Research Trends in Medical Sciences Series

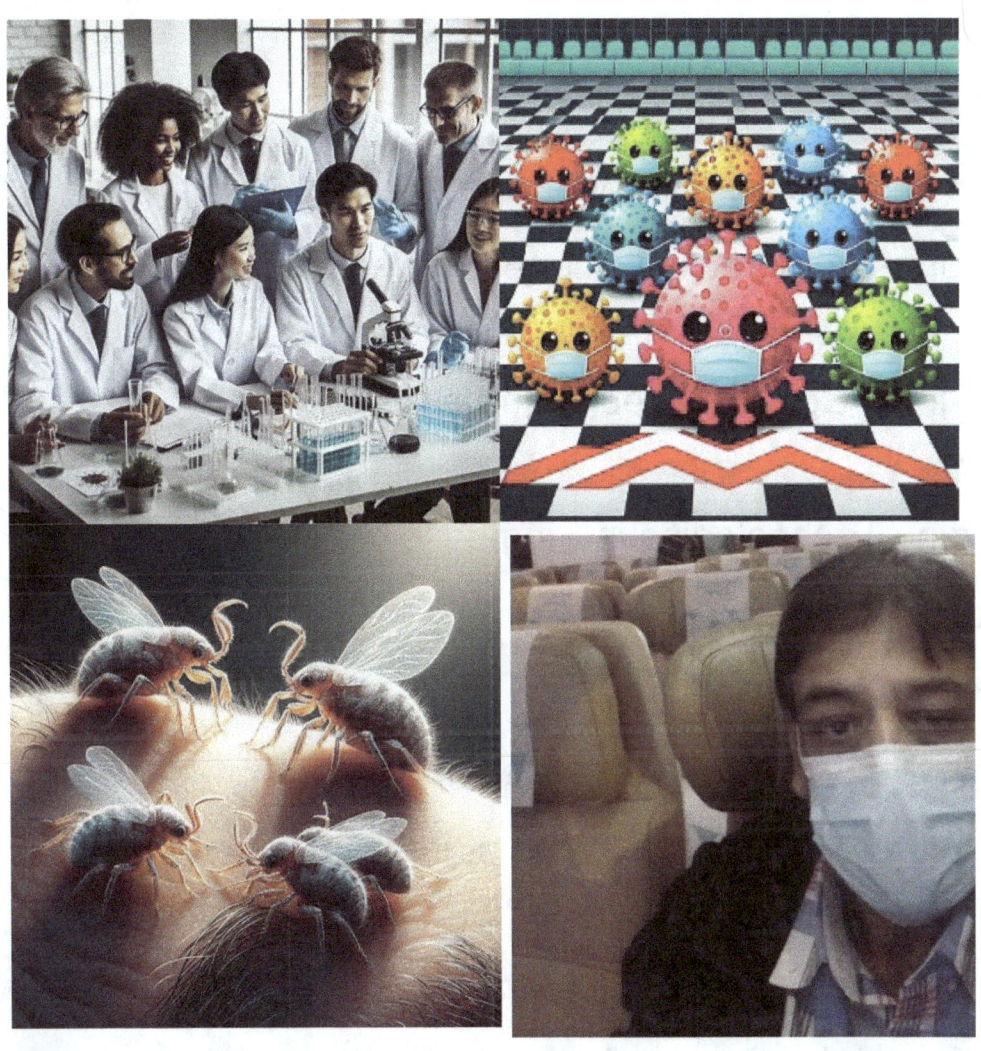

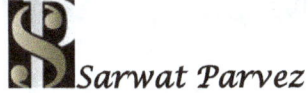Sarwat Parvez

Maryland, USA

Ex Department of Microbiology, PSMMC, Riyadh, Saudi Arabia

Table of Contents

Introduction

The field of medical sciences is witnessing a surge of innovative research trends that promise to reshape our understanding and treatment of various health conditions. One such trend is exploring the brain's structure, which is now understood to be in a delicate balance, crucial for maintaining cognitive functions. Advances in single-cell RNA sequencing techniques are revolutionizing our ability to study individual cells in unprecedented detail, opening new avenues for personalized medicine. Concurrently, protein studies are at the forefront of developing new antibiotics, addressing the growing concern of antibiotic resistance. Insights into chronic Hepatitis E infection are leading to better diagnostic and treatment strategies, enhancing patient care. The use of lung organoids has become instrumental in revealing the strategies pathogens use to invade and infect, which is critical in the fight against respiratory diseases. The quest for next-generation antibiotics is gaining momentum, with researchers unlocking new compounds that could lead to more effective treatments. Green chemistry is expanding within the pharmaceutical industry, promoting sustainability and reducing environmental impact. The clinical validation of CRISPR technology marks a significant milestone, offering hope for curing genetic disorders. The rise of biomaterials is leading to the development of more biocompatible medical devices and implants, improving patient outcomes. Lastly, there is significant progress in treating 'undruggable' diseases, with new drugs targeting previously inaccessible molecular pathways. These trends highlight the dynamic and transformative nature of medical research, holding great promise for the future of healthcare.

Brain's Structure Hangs in 'a Delicate Balance':

Researchers have examined the anatomy of neurons from humans, mice, and fruit flies. They discovered that the cellular structure of the brain is at a critical point, poised between two phases. These new insights could help design computational models of the brain's function.

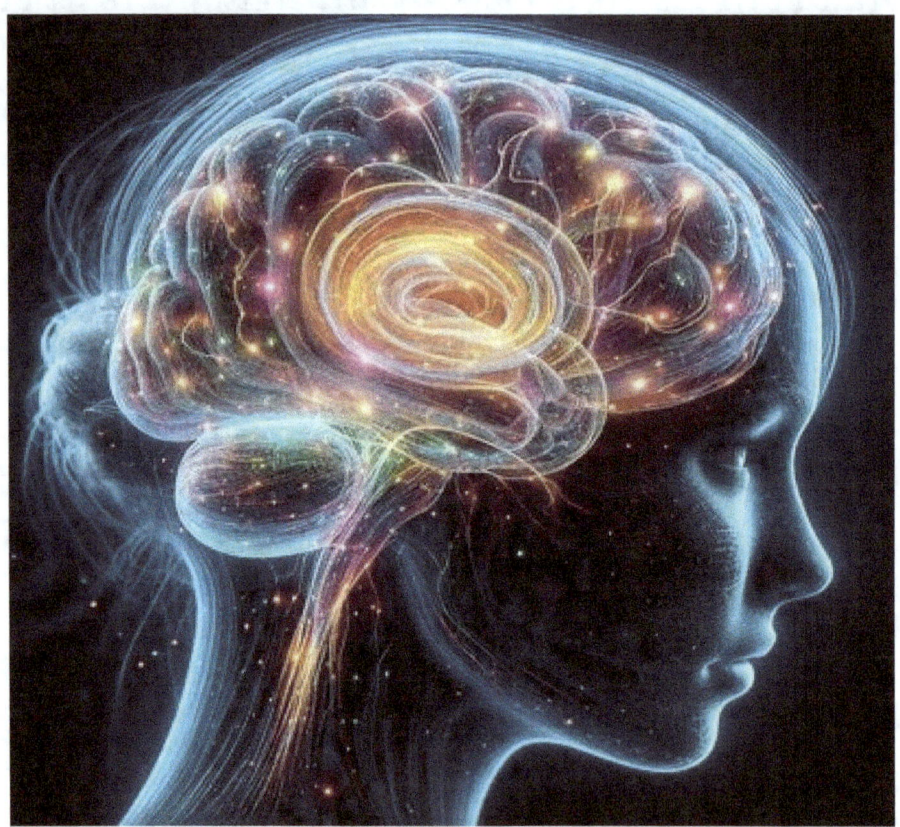

The intricate architecture of the brain, a subject of fascination and study for scientists over the years, has revealed a new layer of complexity. A recent study has shown that the brain's structure is delicately balanced at a critical point, akin to the precise moment of equilibrium before water shifts from solid to liquid.

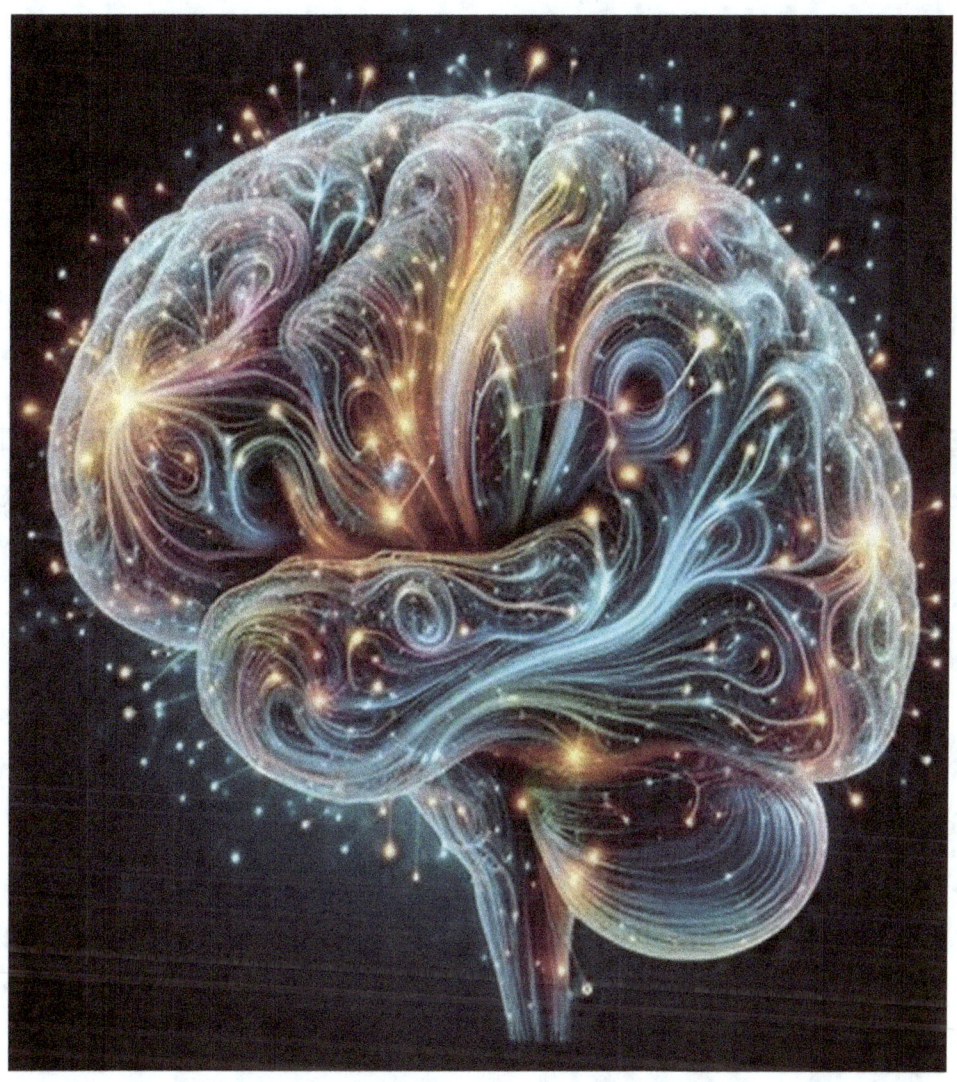

This discovery, consistent across species from humans to fruit flies, suggests a universal principle at work in the organization of neural tissue. At this critical juncture, the brain's structure is neither too rigid nor too fluid, allowing for the dynamic and complex behaviors associated with thought, memory, and consciousness. Understanding this balance could revolutionize our approach to creating computational models that mimic the brain's processing abilities, potentially leading to breakthroughs in artificial intelligence and neurological medicine. The implications of such a finding are profound, as it could mean that the brain operates at a state of optimal complexity, necessary for the emergent properties that underlie cognitive functions. This balance might be what allows the brain to adapt and respond to the myriads of stimuli it encounters, supporting the fluidity of thought and the robustness of memory. As researchers delve deeper into the structural criticality of the brain, they may uncover new strategies for treating neurological disorders, enhancing cognitive function, and even understanding the essence of consciousness itself. The study, a collaborative effort that bridges neuroscience and physics, offers a tantalizing glimpse into the fundamental nature of one of the most complex known systems: the human brain.

Brain's measurement of the critical point involves a multifaceted approach, combining advanced imaging techniques and computational analysis. Researchers utilize tools like functional magnetic resonance imaging (fMRI) and electroencephalograms (EEG) to study brain dynamics and gather massive datasets regarding the brain's cellular structure.

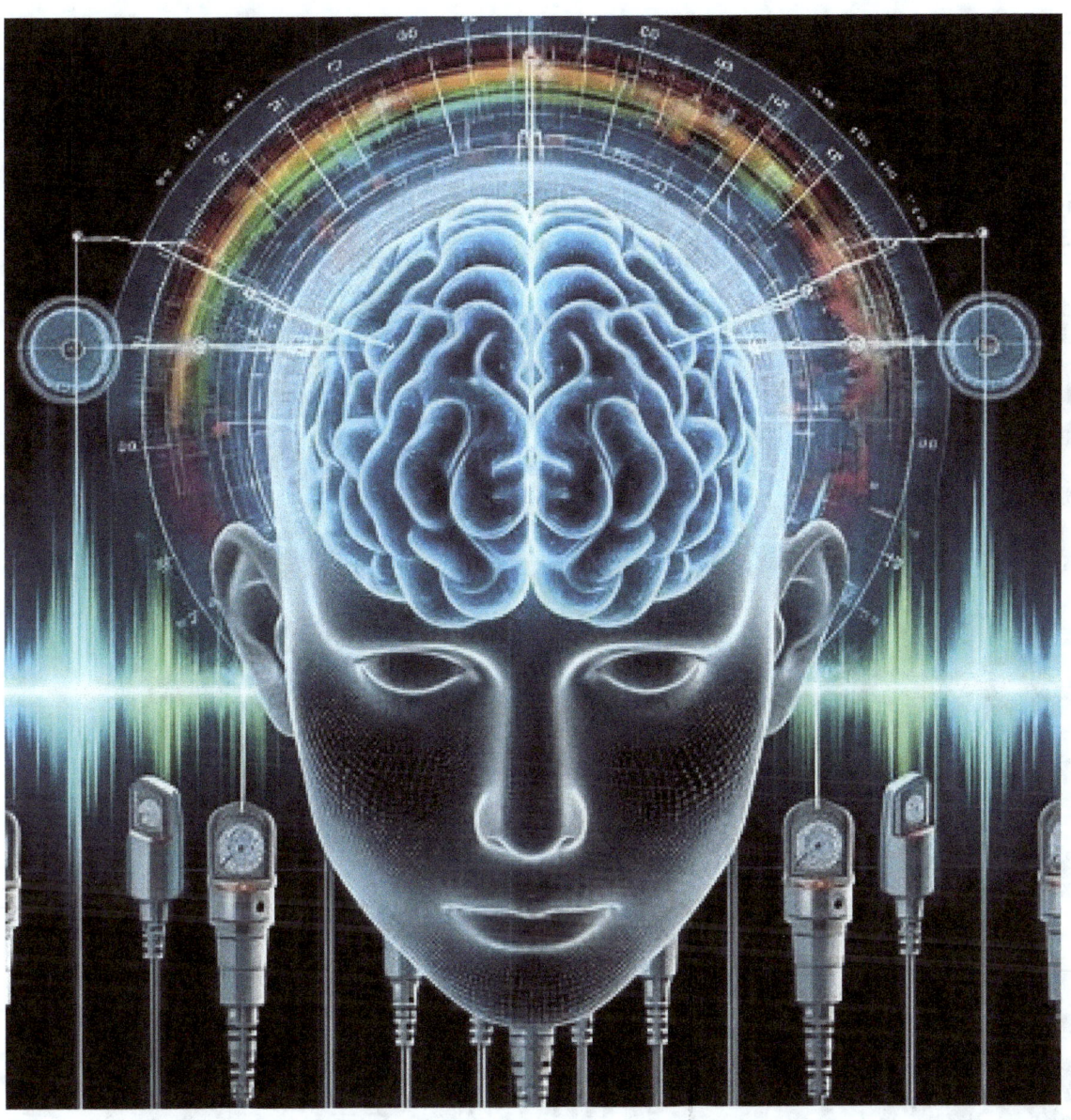

These datasets are then analyzed to identify patterns that suggest the brain is near a phase transition, a state of high complexity where the system is transitioning smoothly from one phase to another. This concept of criticality is borrowed from physics, where it describes the point at which a material changes state, such as a magnet losing its magnetization when heated. In the context of the brain, scientists are investigating the structural level of neurons to understand how this underpins the complexity of brain dynamics. The research suggests that the brain operates at a state of optimal complexity, necessary for cognitive functions like thought and memory. By examining the anatomy of neurons and the way they are organized, researchers can infer the presence of a critical point, which is indicative of the brain's ability to adapt and respond to stimuli with robustness and fluidity.

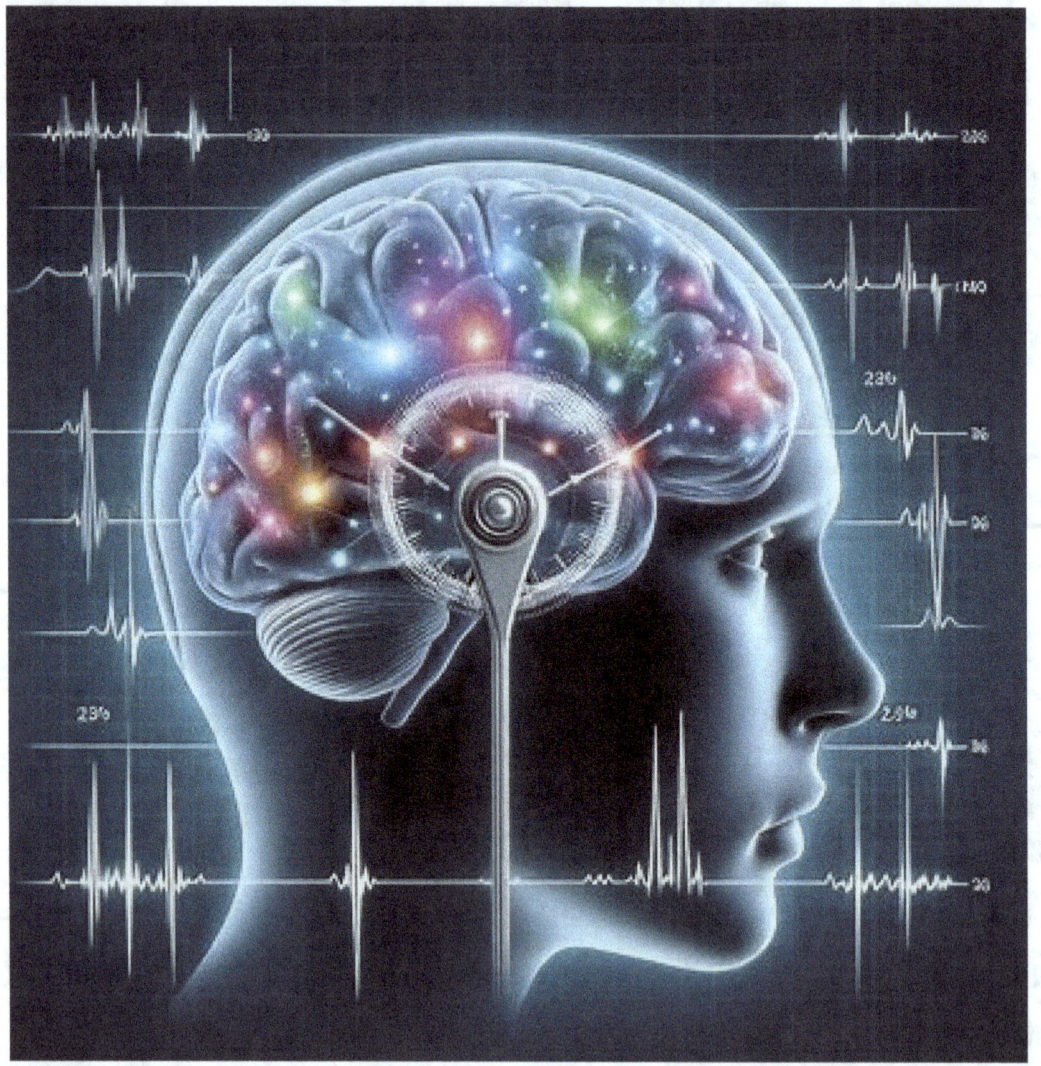

To explore the complexities of the brain's structure, scientists employ a variety of sophisticated techniques. Beyond the commonly known methods such as functional magnetic resonance imaging (fMRI) and electroencephalography (EEG), there are several other advanced tools. Computerized tomography (CT) scans, for instance, provide cross-sectional images of the brain using X-rays, which can be useful for detecting structural changes or abnormalities. Positron emission tomography (PET) scans go a step further by measuring metabolic processes, offering insights into the brain's function by tracking the movement of a radioactive tracer in the brain.

Another intriguing method is magnetoencephalography (MEG), which captures the magnetic fields produced by neural activity, providing a real-time view of brain function. Similarly, functional near-infrared spectroscopy (fNIRS) measures brain activity by detecting changes in blood flow, using infrared light to assess the brain's oxygenation levels. These imaging techniques are non-invasive and have revolutionized our understanding of the brain's structure and function.

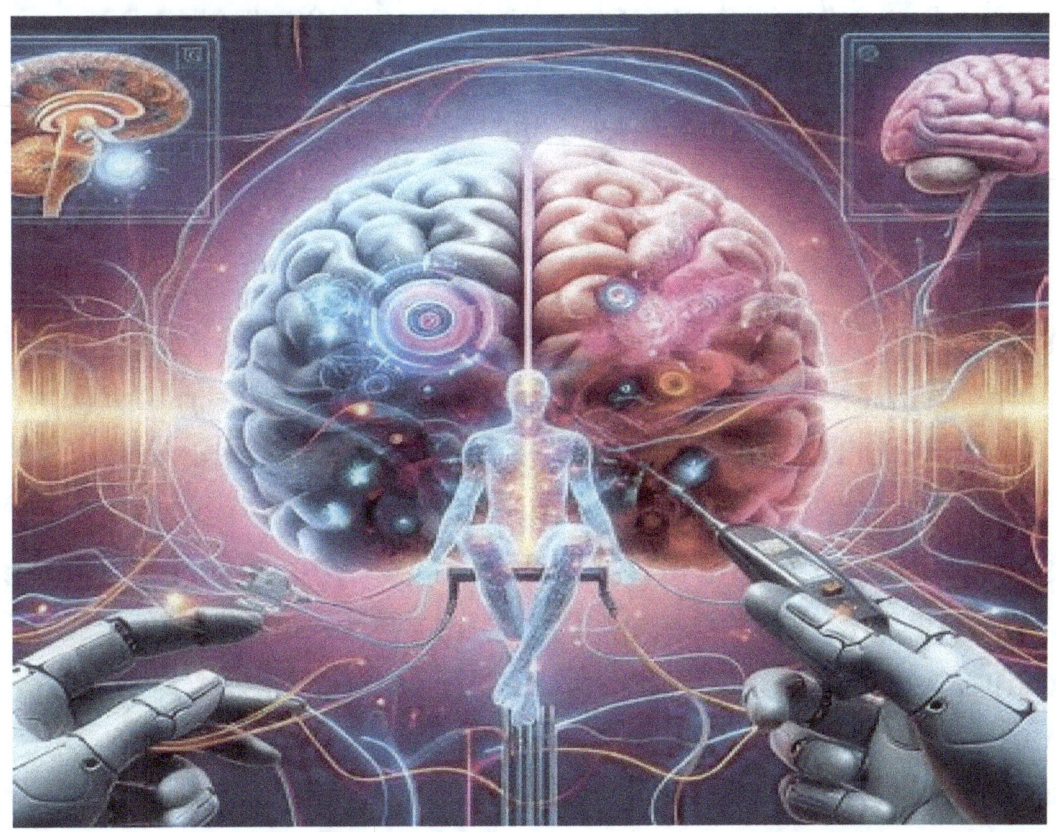

Researchers also study the brain post-mortem, which allows for a detailed examination of the brain's anatomy. This method has provided invaluable insights, especially when comparing healthy brains to those affected by various neurological conditions. Lesions, which can occur naturally due to strokes or injuries, or be induced for research purposes, offer a unique perspective on brain function by highlighting what capabilities are lost when specific areas are damaged.

In addition to imaging, scientists use a range of molecular and genetic tools to study brain structure at the cellular level. Techniques like single-cell RNA sequencing allow for the examination of gene expression patterns in individual neurons, shedding light on the molecular underpinnings of brain function and structure. Advanced microscopy techniques, including electron microscopy, provide ultra-high-resolution images of brain tissue, enabling the study of synaptic connections and neuronal networks with unprecedented detail.

The integration of these diverse techniques, each with its own strengths, is crucial for a comprehensive understanding of the brain. By combining structural imaging with functional and molecular analyses, researchers can correlate the physical architecture of the brain with its dynamic activities and cognitive functions. This multidisciplinary approach is essential for unraveling the mysteries of the brain and could lead to new treatments for neurological disorders, as well as advancements in artificial intelligence that mimic the brain's processing capabilities. The ongoing development of these techniques promises to deepen our knowledge of the brain's intricate structure and how it relates to the vast array of behaviors and mental processes that define human experience.

Single Cell RNA Technique

Single-cell RNA sequencing (scRNA-seq) is a revolutionary technique that allows researchers to examine the gene expression profiles of individual cells. This method has transformed our understanding of the complexity and diversity of cells within tissues and organs. The process begins with the isolation of single cells from a biological sample, which can be achieved through various methods such as fluorescence-activated cell sorting (FACS), microfluidics, or manual picking. Once isolated, the RNA from each cell is reverse transcribed to create complementary DNA (cDNA). This cDNA is then amplified to generate sufficient material for sequencing.

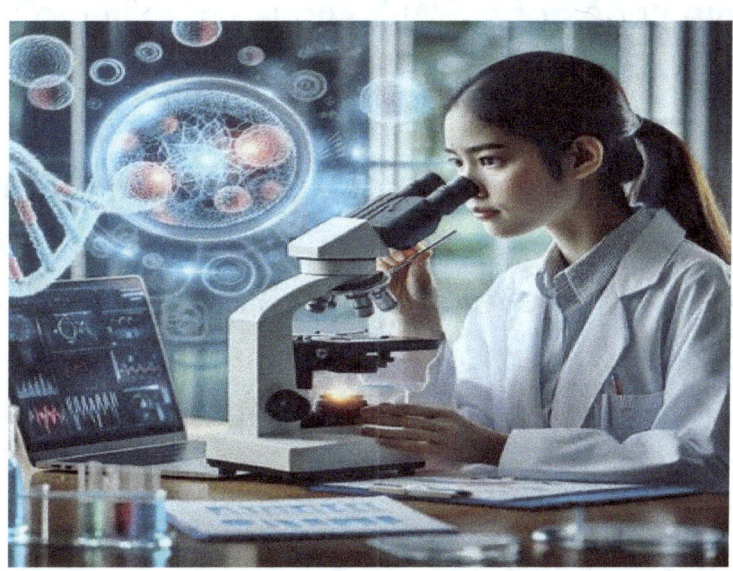

The amplified cDNA fragments are tagged with unique molecular identifiers (UMIs), which enable the tracking of individual RNA molecules back to their cell of origin. These tagged fragments are then sequenced using high-throughput next-generation sequencing (NGS) platforms. The resulting reads are mapped to a reference genome, providing a count of the number of reads associated with each gene, which serves as a proxy for gene expression levels within that cell.

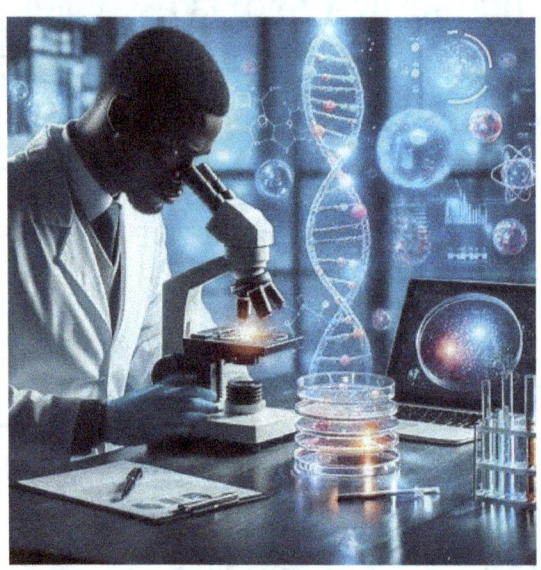

One of the key advantages of scRNA-seq is its ability to uncover cellular heterogeneity within populations that appear homogeneous when analyzed in bulk. This is particularly important in cancer research, where scRNA-seq can identify rare subpopulations of cells that may contribute to disease progression or treatment resistance. In developmental biology, scRNA-seq helps elucidate the trajectories of differentiating cells, shedding light on the processes that lead to the formation of complex tissues.

The data generated by scRNA-seq is rich and multidimensional, requiring sophisticated bioinformatics tools for analysis. Researchers use algorithms to cluster cells based on their gene expression profiles, identify marker genes for different cell types, and infer developmental lineages. These analyses can also reveal gene regulatory networks and pathways that are active in specific cell states.

Despite its power, scRNA-seq comes with technical challenges. The minute amount of RNA in a single cell means that any degradation or loss during preparation can significantly impact the quality of the data. Amplification steps can introduce biases, and the sensitivity of the technique makes it susceptible to contamination. Moreover, the stochastic nature of gene expression can lead to 'dropout' events, where genes are not detected even though they are expressed.

To address these issues, continuous improvements are being made in scRNA-seq protocols and technologies. Innovations such as droplet-based scRNA-seq have increased throughput and reduced costs, making the technique more accessible. Computational methods are also evolving to better handle the complexity of scRNA-seq data, improving the accuracy of cell-type identification and the interpretation of cellular states.

In conclusion, single-cell RNA sequencing is a powerful tool that provides unprecedented insights into the molecular workings of individual cells. Its applications span across various fields of biology and medicine, offering the potential to unravel the complexities of health and disease at the level of single cells. As technology advances, it promises to continue to revolutionize our understanding of biological systems.

What are some limitations of scRNA-seq?

Single-cell RNA sequencing (scRNA-seq) is a powerful tool for understanding cellular complexity, but it is not without its limitations. One significant challenge is the issue of transcript coverage bias, which can lead to the preferential detection of abundant transcripts over those that are less abundant. This bias can skew the perceived expression levels within a cell, potentially obscuring important biological signals. Another limitation is the sequencing coverage itself; due to the minute amount of RNA present in a single cell, it is difficult to achieve the same depth of coverage as bulk RNA sequencing, which can analyze RNA from millions of cells at once. This lower coverage can result in a higher degree of noise and variability in the data, making it harder to draw definitive conclusions.

Capture efficiency is another hurdle; not all RNA molecules from a cell are captured and sequenced, which can lead to incomplete data and the underrepresentation of certain genes or gene isoforms. This problem is exacerbated by the fact that the efficiency of capture can vary from cell to cell, introducing further variability into the dataset. The sensitivity of scRNA-seq also means that it is prone to contamination, which can come from various sources, including ambient RNA or cross-contamination between samples. Such contamination can introduce artifacts into the data, complicating the analysis.

The amplification step required to generate sufficient cDNA for sequencing can introduce its own biases, as some sequences may be more prone to amplification than others. This can distort the true representation of the RNA in the original cell. Additionally, the stochastic nature of gene expression leads to dropout events, where genes that are expressed in the cell are not detected in the sequencing process. These dropouts can create gaps in the data, making it challenging to reconstruct accurate gene expression profiles.

Technical limitations aside, there are also practical constraints to consider. scRNA-seq experiments can be expensive and labor-intensive, limiting the number of cells that can be realistically sequenced in a study. This can impact the statistical power of the analysis and the ability to detect rare cell types or transient states. The requirement for specialized equipment and expertise can also be a barrier, making scRNA-seq less accessible to all researchers.

Despite these challenges, scRNA-seq remains a valuable method for exploring cellular heterogeneity and the molecular underpinnings of health and disease. Ongoing advancements in technology and computational methods continue to address these limitations, improving the reliability and accessibility of single-cell sequencing data. As the field progresses, it is likely that many of the current limitations will be overcome, further unlocking the potential of scRNA-seq to provide insights into the complexities of biological systems.

How is scRNA-seq different from bulk RNA sequencing?

Single-cell RNA sequencing (scRNA-seq) and bulk RNA sequencing are both powerful techniques used to analyze gene expression, but they differ significantly in their approach and the level of detail they provide. Bulk RNA sequencing analyzes the total RNA from a mixed population of cells, providing an average expression profile for the sample. This method is useful for understanding the overall gene expression patterns in a tissue or cell culture, but it cannot distinguish between the contributions of different cell types or states within the sample. In contrast, scRNA-seq analyzes the RNA content of individual cells, allowing researchers to explore the cellular heterogeneity and identify distinct gene expression profiles at the single-cell level.

The differences between scRNA-seq and bulk RNA sequencing extend to their technical aspects as well. scRNA-seq requires the isolation of single cells, which can be challenging and requires specialized equipment. The technique also involves capturing and amplifying the RNA from each cell separately, which can introduce technical variability. However, this single-cell resolution enables the identification of rare cell types and the characterization of complex tissues, which would be impossible with bulk sequencing.

In terms of data analysis, scRNA-seq generates large datasets that require advanced bioinformatics tools to interpret. The data from each cell must be analyzed individually, which can be computationally intensive. Bulk RNA sequencing data is generally simpler to analyze because it represents an average of all cells in the sample. However, this averaging can mask the contributions of rare cell types and subtle changes in gene expression that are critical for understanding complex biological processes.

Another key difference is the application of each technique. scRNA-seq is particularly useful in research areas where cellular heterogeneity plays a significant role, such as in cancer, where it can reveal the presence of different tumor cell subpopulations. Bulk RNA sequencing is often used in situations where the overall gene expression pattern is of interest, such as in response to a drug treatment in a cell culture model.

In summary, while both scRNA-seq and bulk RNA sequencing are valuable tools for gene expression analysis, they serve different purposes and provide different levels of insight into the biology of cells and tissues. scRNA-seq offers a high-resolution view of cellular diversity, while bulk RNA sequencing provides a broader overview of gene expression across a population of cells. The choice between the two methods depends on the specific research questions and the level of detail required.

What are some practical scenarios where bulk RNA sequencing is more appropriate?

Bulk RNA sequencing is particularly advantageous in scenarios where the primary goal is to obtain a general overview of gene expression across many cells or when the sample size is too small for individual cell isolation. This method is cost-effective for generating large amounts of data, making it suitable for projects with limited budgets or resources. It is also the method of choice when working with complex tissues or organisms where cell types cannot be easily separated, such as in the case of solid tumors or integrated organ tissues.

In developmental biology, bulk RNA sequencing can be used to track gene expression changes over time, providing insights into the dynamic processes of development and differentiation. It is also useful in pharmacogenomics, where researchers are interested in the overall response of tissues or cell cultures to drug treatments, rather than the responses of individual cells. In agricultural research, bulk RNA sequencing helps study plants' genetic responses to environmental stressors, pests, or diseases, which is critical for crop improvement and sustainability efforts.

Moreover, bulk RNA sequencing is beneficial in studies aiming to compare gene expression between different conditions, such as healthy versus diseased states, across large patient cohorts. This approach can identify biomarkers and therapeutic targets by highlighting genes that are consistently upregulated or downregulated in a disease context. In neuroscience, bulk RNA sequencing can be used to analyze the global gene expression patterns in different regions of the brain, contributing to our understanding of brain function and the molecular basis of neurological disorders.

In the field of immunology, bulk RNA sequencing can assess the overall immune response by analyzing gene expression in blood samples or lymphoid tissues. This is particularly relevant in the study of systemic diseases or when monitoring the immune response to infections or vaccinations. Additionally, bulk RNA sequencing is useful in conservation biology, where it can be applied to study the genetic diversity and adaptive responses of endangered species to environmental changes.

In cancer research, while single-cell sequencing is invaluable for understanding tumor heterogeneity, bulk RNA sequencing is still widely used for initial screenings to identify key pathways and genes involved in tumorigenesis. It serves as a preliminary step before more detailed single-cell analyses are conducted. Bulk RNA sequencing is also employed in transcriptome-wide association studies (TWAS), which correlate gene expression levels with genetic variants to identify genes associated with complex traits and diseases.

Lastly, bulk RNA sequencing is appropriate in situations where the cellular composition of the sample is known and uniform, such as in cell lines or clonal populations. In these cases, the averaging effect of bulk sequencing is not a disadvantage but rather provides a clear and concise expression profile of the population.

In summary, bulk RNA sequencing remains a valuable tool in genomics research, offering a cost-effective and efficient way to analyze gene expression patterns across a wide range of biological samples and experimental conditions. Its applications are diverse, spanning from basic research to clinical studies, and it continues to provide fundamental insights into the molecular mechanisms underlying various biological processes and diseases.

Validating bulk RNA sequencing results is a critical step in ensuring the accuracy and reliability of gene expression data. Researchers employ several strategies to confirm that their sequencing results reflect true biological signals rather than technical artifacts or random noise. One common approach is the use of technical replicates, where the same sample is sequenced multiple times to assess the consistency of the results. This helps to identify and account for any variability introduced by the sequencing process itself.

Another method is the comparison of RNA sequencing results with those obtained from other established techniques, such as quantitative PCR (qPCR). qPCR is considered a gold standard for measuring gene expression due to its high sensitivity and specificity. By comparing RNA-seq data to qPCR results for a subset of genes, researchers can validate the expression patterns observed in their sequencing experiments.

Cross-validation with independent datasets is also a valuable technique. Researchers can compare their results with publicly available RNA-seq datasets from similar experiments or conditions. This not only provides a form of external validation but also helps to put the findings in a broader context, enhancing the overall robustness of the conclusions drawn from the data.

Bioinformatics tools play a crucial role in the validation process as well. Software like DESeq2, edgeR, or limma can be used to perform differential gene expression analysis, which identifies genes that are significantly upregulated or downregulated between different conditions or treatments. These analyses include statistical tests that help to determine the likelihood that the observed changes in gene expression are due to chance.

Quality control metrics are another essential aspect of validation. Measures such as the RNA Integrity Number (RIN) and DV200, which assess the integrity and quality of the RNA samples, are crucial for interpreting the reliability of RNA-seq data. High-quality RNA is more likely to yield accurate and reproducible results, so ensuring the RNA meets certain standards before sequencing is a key step in the validation process.

Normalization of the data is also important to account for differences in sequencing depth and to correct for batch effects, which can arise from variations in sample processing or sequencing runs. Tools like ComBat, CombatSeq, or MNN are specifically designed to correct for these batch effects, ensuring that the results are not skewed by technical discrepancies.

In addition to these methods, spike-in controls, which are known quantities of RNA from an external source, can be added to the samples before sequencing. The consistency of the spike-in controls across different samples can serve as a benchmark for the accuracy of the RNA-seq data. This approach is particularly useful for adjusting for variations in library preparation and sequencing efficiency.

Finally, integrated analysis of single-cell and bulk RNA sequencing data can provide a comprehensive view of gene expression. By comparing the results from bulk RNA-seq with those from single-cell sequencing, researchers can validate the expression patterns observed at the population level against the more detailed resolution provided by single-cell analysis. This can be especially informative in studies of heterogeneous samples, such as tumors, where the bulk data may mask the contributions of distinct cell populations.

In summary, validating bulk RNA sequencing results involves a combination of experimental and computational approaches. Technical replicates, cross-validation with other techniques and datasets, bioinformatics analyses, quality control metrics, normalization procedures, spike-in controls, and integrated analyses with single-cell data all contribute to the robustness and credibility of RNA-seq experiments. These validation steps are essential for ensuring that the gene expression profiles obtained from RNA-seq accurately reflect the underlying biology of the samples being studied.

RNA-seq data analysis is a complex process that can be fraught with potential pitfalls, which can lead to inaccurate conclusions if not properly addressed. One common issue is the quality of RNA samples; degraded RNA can significantly affect the accuracy of sequencing results. Ensuring high-quality, intact RNA is crucial for reliable data. Another pitfall is the choice of sequencing depth and coverage. Insufficient sequencing depth may result in missing lowly expressed genes, while excessive depth can be cost-inefficient without adding significant value to the analysis.

The alignment of reads to the reference genome or transcriptome is another critical step where errors can occur. Incorrect alignment can lead to false gene expression levels. It's essential to use updated and accurate reference sequences and to consider the possibility of alternative splicing events. Similarly, the choice of bioinformatics tools and parameters for read mapping and quantification can greatly influence the results. Different tools and settings can yield varying outcomes, so it's important to select the most appropriate ones for the specific study design and to validate the chosen methods.

Normalization of data is a key step in RNA-seq analysis to account for technical variations. Failure to properly normalize data can lead to misleading differential expression results.

Researchers must choose suitable normalization methods that fit their data characteristics and experimental design. Batch effects are another source of error, where non-biological differences between samples can skew results. Proper experimental design and statistical methods are required to identify and correct batch effects.

The statistical analysis of RNA-seq data also presents challenges. The use of inappropriate statistical tests or failure to adjust for multiple tests can result in false positives or negatives. It's vital to apply rigorous statistical frameworks that are tailored to the distribution and nature of RNA-seq data. Interpretation of results is another area where pitfalls can occur. Overinterpretation of small changes in gene expression or disregarding biological relevance can lead to incorrect conclusions. Researchers must critically evaluate their results in the context of biological systems and existing literature.

In single-cell RNA-seq (scRNA-seq), additional complexities arise. The sparsity of the data, where many genes are not detected in individual cells, requires specialized computational approaches. Dropout events, where true gene expression is not captured, can complicate the analysis and interpretation of scRNA-seq data. The heterogeneity of cell populations also poses challenges; distinguishing between true biological variation and technical noise is essential for accurate characterization of cell types and states.

Finally, reproducibility is a concern in RNA-seq analysis. Without clear documentation of the analysis pipeline and parameters, it can be difficult for other researchers to replicate the study. Ensuring that the analysis is transparent and reproducible is critical for the credibility and utility of the results. By being aware of these common pitfalls and taking steps to address them, researchers can improve the accuracy and reliability of their RNA-seq data analysis, leading to more robust scientific findings.

How Single Cell RNA Technique can be made Cost-effective?

Making single-cell RNA sequencing (scRNA-seq) more cost-effective is a multifaceted challenge that requires strategic planning and innovation at various stages of the workflow. One approach is to optimize the experimental design to ensure that the number of cells sequenced aligns with the study's objectives, avoiding unnecessary sequencing that can inflate costs. Researchers can also consider pooling samples or using multiplexing techniques, which allow for the simultaneous processing of multiple samples, thereby reducing reagent costs and minimizing technical variability.

Advancements in microfluidics and the development of in-house protocols for reagent preparation can also contribute to cost reductions. Microfluidic devices can decrease the volume of reagents required, and in-house protocols can replace more expensive commercial kits. Additionally, the use of UMIs (Unique Molecular Identifiers) can improve the accuracy of quantification and reduce the sequencing depth needed, further lowering sequencing costs.

Another strategy is to leverage computational methods to maximize the information extracted from the data. For instance, bioinformatics tools can help identify the optimal number of reads per cell, balancing the depth of sequencing with the project's budget constraints. The use of open-source software for data analysis can also eliminate the need for costly proprietary software licenses.

Collaborations and shared resources, such as core facilities or consortium projects, can provide access to scRNA-seq technologies at a lower individual cost. By sharing the expenses associated with high-throughput sequencing equipment and technical expertise, researchers can benefit from economies of scale. Furthermore, the adoption of newer, more efficient sequencing platforms can increase throughput and reduce per-sample costs over time.

In terms of data handling, efficient storage and management of the large datasets generated by scRNA-seq are essential. Investing in data compression and optimization techniques can save on long-term data storage costs, which can be substantial given the size of scRNA-seq datasets. Additionally, careful planning of data analysis pipelines to streamline processing can reduce computational costs.

Educational initiatives and training can also play a role in making scRNA-seq more cost-effective. By increasing the skill level of researchers and technicians in scRNA-seq methodologies, institutions can reduce the reliance on external services and perform more procedures in-house, which can be more economical in the long run.

Lastly, the field can benefit from the development of new technologies and methods that reduce costs. Innovations in sequencing chemistries, library preparation methods, and automation can all contribute to making scRNA-seq more accessible and affordable. As technology matures and competition increases, it is likely that the costs associated with single-cell sequencing will continue to decrease, making it a more viable option for a wider range of research applications. The collective effort to refine and improve scRNA-seq will not only make it more cost-effective but also expand its potential to uncover the complexities of biology at the single-cell level.

Emerging Technologies in Single-Cell RNA Techniques

Emerging technologies in single-cell RNA sequencing (scRNA-seq) are rapidly advancing the field, offering new insights into cellular complexity and gene expression dynamics. Recent developments include droplet-based and plate-based methods, which have significantly increased the throughput and reduced the cost of scRNA-seq. Droplet-based techniques, such as those developed by 10x Genomics, encapsulate individual cells in microfluidic droplets, allowing for the parallel processing of thousands of cells in a single run. Plate-based methods, on the other hand, use microwell plates to isolate and process single cells, providing a more controlled environment for cell capture and analysis.

Hydrogel-based scRNA-seq is another innovative approach that uses hydrogels to encapsulate and barcode individual cells or nuclei. This method can preserve spatial information and enable the study of cell-cell interactions and microenvironments. Spatial transcriptomics is a particularly exciting advancement that combines scRNA-seq with imaging techniques to map gene expression in tissue sections. This technology allows researchers to visualize the spatial distribution of different cell types and their gene expression patterns within the context of their native tissue architecture.

Single-nucleus RNA sequencing (snRNA-seq) is an adaptation of scRNA-seq that sequences RNA from isolated nuclei instead of whole cells. This technique is especially useful for tissues that are difficult to dissociate or for samples where cell viability is a concern. snRNA-seq can provide insights into the transcriptional activity of cells that are otherwise inaccessible to traditional scRNA-seq methods.

Deep learning methods, such as autoencoders and generative adversarial networks (GANs), are emerging as powerful tools for analyzing scRNA-seq data. These computational techniques can help to identify complex patterns in gene expression data, correct for technical noise, and even predict cellular responses to different stimuli. The integration of scRNA-seq with other omics technologies, such as proteomics and metabolomics, is also an area of active development. This multi-omics approach can provide a more comprehensive view of cellular function and the regulatory networks that govern cell behavior.

In addition to these technological advancements, improvements in bioinformatics analysis are crucial for interpreting the vast amounts of data generated by scRNA-seq. New algorithms and software tools are being developed to handle the unique challenges of single-cell data, such as sparsity, noise, and batch effects. These tools are essential for clustering cells, identifying cell types, inferring developmental trajectories, and understanding the molecular mechanisms underlying cellular processes.

The future of scRNA-seq technology lies in further increasing the throughput, reducing costs, and enhancing the resolution of single-cell analysis. Innovations in sample preparation, sequencing chemistries, and data analysis will continue to push the boundaries of what is possible with scRNA-seq. As these emerging technologies mature, they will undoubtedly unlock new discoveries in biology and medicine, shedding light on the intricacies of life at the single-cell level. The ongoing evolution of scRNA-seq technologies promises to deepen our understanding of cellular heterogeneity and the dynamics of gene expression, with profound implications for research in stem cell biology, cancer, neuroscience, developmental biology, and beyond. The integration of scRNA-seq with other cutting-edge technologies will accelerate the pace of discovery and pave the way for novel therapeutic interventions and precision medicine approaches. The potential of scRNA-seq to revolutionize our understanding of complex biological systems is immense, and the continued innovation in this field will be a key driver of scientific progress in the years to come.

Choosing the most suitable single-cell RNA sequencing (scRNA-seq) method for a study involves careful consideration of several key factors. Researchers must first clearly define their research objectives, as different scRNA-seq methods may vary in their ability to detect rare cell types, resolve cell states, or capture the dynamics of gene expression. The nature of the sample is also crucial; some methods are better suited for tissues that are difficult to dissociate, while others may be optimized for blood or cultured cells.

Throughput and scalability are important considerations, especially in studies requiring the analysis of large numbers of cells. High-throughput methods can process thousands of cells simultaneously but may come at a higher cost or with a trade-off in resolution. Conversely, methods with lower throughput might provide higher resolution or sensitivity, which could be critical for detecting lowly expressed genes.

The quality of data generated by the scRNA-seq method is another vital aspect. This includes the level of technical noise, the sensitivity to detect gene expression, and the accuracy of capturing the full transcriptome of each cell. Some methods may offer higher sensitivity but at an increased complexity and cost of data analysis.

Flexibility and compatibility with downstream analyses are also important. The chosen method should be compatible with the available bioinformatics pipelines and should allow for the integration of data with other omics datasets if necessary. Additionally, the method should be adaptable to future technological advancements and research questions.

Cost-effectiveness is a practical concern that cannot be overlooked. While some scRNA-seq methods may offer superior data quality, they may also be prohibitively expensive for some research budgets. Researchers must balance the cost with the expected outcome and the potential for funding.

Lastly, the technical expertise available and the infrastructure of the research facility can influence the choice of scRNA-seq method. Some methods require specialized equipment and trained personnel, which may not be available in all research settings. It's essential to consider the technical and logistical capabilities of the research team and facility when selecting a method.

In summary, selecting the most suitable scRNA-seq method is a multifaceted decision that depends on the specific goals and constraints of the research project. Researchers must weigh the trade-offs between data quality, throughput, cost, and technical requirements to choose the method that best aligns with their study's needs. Consulting with experts in the field, reviewing the latest literature, and considering the long-term goals of the research are all part of making an informed decision. The choice of scRNA-seq method can significantly impact the study's outcomes, so it is a decision that warrants thorough consideration and planning. By carefully evaluating the available options and aligning them with the study's objectives and resources, researchers can maximize the potential of scRNA-seq to yield meaningful and impactful scientific insights. The ongoing advancements in scRNA-seq technologies continue to expand the range of available methods, providing researchers with an ever-growing toolkit to explore the complexities of biology at the single-cell level. As the field evolves, the criteria for selecting a scRNA-seq method may also change, emphasizing the importance of staying informed about the latest developments and best practices in single-cell genomics. The goal is to select a scRNA-seq method that not only meets the immediate needs of the study but also positions the research for future discoveries and applications. With careful planning and consideration, scRNA-seq can be a powerful approach to uncovering the intricacies of cellular function and gene expression, driving forward our understanding of health and disease.

Challenges

Single-cell RNA sequencing (scRNA-seq) has revolutionized the field of genomics by providing insights at a resolution that was previously unattainable. However, designing a scRNA-seq experiment is a complex task that comes with several challenges. One of the primary concerns is ensuring the quality and viability of the starting material, as the condition of the cells can significantly impact the results. Cell isolation techniques must be optimized to maintain cell integrity while minimizing stress and cell death, which can alter gene expression profiles.

Another challenge is the selection of an appropriate scRNA-seq platform, as different technologies can vary in terms of throughput, sensitivity, and cost. Researchers must balance these factors against their specific research questions and the expected cell heterogeneity within their samples. The issue of capturing enough cells to represent rare cell populations is also critical, especially in heterogeneous samples like tumors or developing tissues. This requires careful planning to ensure that the sample size is sufficient to detect and analyze these rare cell types.

Technical variability is another hurdle in scRNA-seq experimental design. This includes batch effects, which can arise from differences in cell handling, reagent lots, or sequencing runs.

Such variability must be accounted for in the experimental design and data analysis to avoid confounding biological interpretations. The presence of ambient RNA, resulting from cell lysis or other sources, can also introduce noise into the data, necessitating rigorous quality control measures.

The high sensitivity of scRNA-seq can lead to the detection of 'dropouts,' where genes are not detected even though they are expressed. This can be due to technical issues like inefficient mRNA capture or reverse transcription, or biological factors such as low gene expression levels. Addressing dropouts is essential for accurate data interpretation and often requires sophisticated computational tools.

Data analysis poses its own set of challenges, as scRNA-seq data is typically sparse and noisy. The development and application of robust bioinformatics pipelines are crucial for data processing, normalization, and analysis. Researchers must also contend with the computational demands of handling large datasets, which can be resource intensive.

Ethical considerations are increasingly important in scRNA-seq experimental design, particularly when human samples are involved. Ensuring patient consent and data privacy is paramount, and researchers must navigate the regulatory landscape carefully to comply with ethical standards.

In conclusion, scRNA-seq experimental design is a multifaceted process that requires careful consideration of technical, biological, and ethical factors. Addressing these challenges is essential for generating high-quality data that can lead to meaningful biological insights. As technology continues to evolve, so will the strategies for overcoming these obstacles, enabling researchers to harness the full potential of scRNA-seq in their studies. The ongoing dialogue between technologists, biologists, and bioinformaticians is crucial for the development of best practices in scRNA-seq experimental design, ensuring that this powerful technique continues to advance our understanding of complex biological systems. The collective effort to refine and improve scRNA-seq methodologies will not only enhance the quality of the data but also expand the scope of research questions that can be addressed, paving the way for new discoveries in the field of genomics. The challenges in scRNA-seq experimental design are significant, but they are not insurmountable. With continued innovation and collaboration, researchers can overcome these hurdles and unlock the full potential of single-cell analysis. The future of scRNA-seq is bright, and the insights gained from these studies will undoubtedly have a profound impact on our understanding of biology and disease. The commitment to excellence in experimental design is what will drive the field forward, ensuring that scRNA-seq remains at the forefront of genomic research. The dedication to overcoming the challenges of scRNA-seq experimental design reflects the broader scientific pursuit of knowledge and the desire to push the boundaries of what is possible. Through this pursuit, scRNA-seq will continue to illuminate the intricacies of life at the single-cell level, offering a window into the diversity and dynamism of cellular life. The journey of discovery is just beginning, and the challenges in scRNA-seq experimental design are but steppingstones on the path to greater understanding. The quest for knowledge is a driving force in science, and scRNA-seq is a powerful tool in this quest. As researchers rise to meet the challenges of experimental design, they pave the way for future generations of scientists to explore the uncharted territories of the cellular landscape. The challenges are many, but the rewards are great, and the pursuit of knowledge through scRNA-seq is a worthy endeavor that will continue to inspire and inform the scientific community for years to come. The spirit of inquiry and the determination to overcome obstacles are what define the scientific endeavor, and scRNA-seq is a testament to the relentless pursuit of understanding that characterizes the field of genomics. The challenges in experimental design are but a part of the larger journey of discovery, and with each challenge overcome, the field of scRNA-seq moves one step closer to unlocking the secrets of cellular life. The path forward is paved with challenges, but it is also lined with the promise of discovery, and the scientific community stands ready to meet these challenges head-on. The future of scRNA-seq is a future of possibility, and the challenges in experimental design are the gateways to new frontiers in genomic research. The commitment to overcoming these challenges is a commitment to the advancement of science, and the rewards of this commitment are the insights and discoveries that will shape our understanding of the world around us. The challenges in scRNA-seq experimental design are a call to action for the scientific community, a reminder that there is always more to learn, and that the pursuit of knowledge is an ever-evolving journey. The field of scRNA-seq is a field of opportunity, and the challenges in experimental design are opportunities for growth, innovation, and discovery. The scientific community's response to these challenges will define the future of scRNA-seq, and the future is bright with the promise of new knowledge and understanding. The journey of scRNA-seq is a journey of exploration, and the challenges in experimental design are milestones along the way. With each challenge overcome, the field of scRNA-seq advances, bringing new insights and new understanding to the forefront of genomic research. The challenges are many, but the spirit of discovery is strong, and the field of scRNA-seq will continue to thrive as researchers rise to meet these challenges with determination and ingenuity. The path ahead is filled with challenges, but it is also filled with potential, and the field of scRNA-seq stands poised to unlock the mysteries of cellular life, one cell at a time. The challenges in experimental design are the steppingstones to a future of discovery, and the scientific community is ready to take the next step. The future of scRNA-seq is a future of exploration, and the challenges in experimental design are the compass points guiding the way. With each challenge navigated, the field of scRNA-seq charts a course toward a deeper understanding of the cellular world, and the scientific community follows this course with anticipation and excitement. The challenges in scRNA-seq experimental design are the sparks that ignite the flame of discovery, and the field of scRNA-seq is the torchbearer, leading the way into the unknown. The journey is long, but the destination is worth the effort, and the field of scRNA-seq is on the path to new horizons in genomic research. The challenges in experimental design are the tests of our resolve, and the field of scRNA-seq is rising to the challenge, forging ahead with resilience and vision. The future of scRNA-seq is a future of innovation, and the challenges in experimental design are the catalysts for change. With each challenge met, the field of scRNA-seq evolves, pushing the boundaries of what is known and expanding the limits of what is possible. The challenges in scRNA-seq experimental design are the hurdles to be cleared, and the field of scRNA-seq is leaping forward, reaching new heights in the pursuit of knowledge. The journey of discovery is an ongoing one, and the challenges in experimental design are the landmarks along the way. The field of scRNA-seq is navigating this journey with expertise and enthusiasm, charting a course toward a future rich with discovery and insight. The challenges in scRNA-seq experimental design are the puzzles to be solved, and the field of scRNA-seq is assembling the pieces, constructing a picture of cellular complexity that is more complete and more detailed than ever before. The future of scRNA-seq is a future of progress, and the challenges in experimental design are the steps toward that progress. With each challenge overcome, the field of scRNA-seq moves forward, advancing our understanding of the cellular landscape and enriching our knowledge of life at the single-cell level. The challenges in scRNA-seq experimental design are the opportunities for growth, and the field of scRNA-seq is growing, expanding its reach and deepening its impact on the world of genomics. The journey of scRNA-seq is a journey of discovery, and the challenges in experimental design are the adventures that await. The field of scRNA-seq is embarking on these adventures with curiosity and courage, exploring the vast and varied terrain of the cellular world. The challenges in scRNA-seq experimental design are the invitations to explore, and the field of scRNA-seq is accepting these invitations with open arms, venturing forth into the unknown with a spirit of exploration and a thirst for knowledge. The future of scRNA-seq is a future of discovery, and the challenges in experimental design are the doorways to that discovery. With each challenge opened, the field of scRNA-seq enters new realms of understanding, uncovering the secrets of cellular life and bringing them into the light of scientific inquiry. The challenges in scRNA-seq experimental design are the gateways to innovation, each one presenting an opportunity to refine techniques and expand our understanding of cellular mechanisms. As researchers navigate these challenges, they contribute to a collective knowledge base that benefits the entire scientific community. The intricacies of single-cell analysis demand precision and creativity, pushing scientists to develop novel solutions that can lead to groundbreaking discoveries.

In the face of these challenges, collaboration becomes a powerful tool. Sharing insights and methodologies across labs and disciplines can accelerate the development of new scRNA-seq technologies and analytical strategies. This collaborative spirit is essential in a field as rapidly evolving as genomics, where today's challenge is tomorrow's breakthrough.

Moreover, the challenges of scRNA-seq experimental design underscore the importance of rigorous training and education. As new technologies emerge, equipping researchers with the skills to effectively utilize these tools is paramount. This not only involves technical training but also fostering a mindset that embraces complexity and uncertainty as part of the scientific process.

The dynamic nature of scRNA-seq also means that experimental design must be adaptable. What works today may not be sufficient tomorrow, and researchers must remain agile, ready to adopt new technologies and approaches as they become available. This adaptability is a hallmark of successful scRNA-seq research, reflecting the ever-changing landscape of genomic science.

Furthermore, the challenges in scRNA-seq experimental design are a testament to the field's maturity. As technology has evolved, so too have the questions we ask and the problems we seek to solve. Each challenge met is a step towards a more nuanced understanding of biology, from the fundamentals of gene expression to the complexities of disease pathology.

The pursuit of solutions to these challenges is driven by a fundamental curiosity about the nature of life. scRNA-seq offers a lens through which we can observe the previously unseen, revealing the diversity and dynamism of individual cells. This curiosity fuels the relentless pursuit of knowledge that defines the field of genomics and the broader scientific endeavor.

As researchers rise to meet the challenges of scRNA-seq experimental design, they do so with the knowledge that their work has the potential to make a lasting impact. The insights gleaned from single-cell analysis can inform everything from basic biological research to the development of new therapies for complex diseases.

The challenges in scRNA-seq experimental design are not just obstacles to be overcome; they are catalysts for growth and discovery. They push the boundaries of what is possible, driving innovation and inspiring a new generation of scientists to explore the frontiers of genomic research.

In conclusion, the challenges of scRNA-seq experimental design are integral to the scientific process. They inspire us to ask deeper questions, develop better technologies, and strive for a more comprehensive understanding of the cellular world. As we continue to navigate these challenges, we pave the way for discoveries that will enrich our understanding of biology and improve the human condition. The journey of scRNA-seq is one of constant learning and discovery, and the challenges we face along the way are the milestones that mark our progress in this exciting field.

Emerging Trends

Emerging trends in single-cell RNA sequencing (scRNA-seq) research reflect the rapid evolution of the field, driven by technological advancements and a growing understanding of cellular complexity. One significant trend is the integration of scRNA-seq with other 'omics' technologies, such as proteomics and metabolomics, to provide a more comprehensive view of cellular function. This multi-omics approach allows for the simultaneous analysis of different molecular layers, offering deeper insights into the regulatory networks that govern cell behavior.

Another trend is the development of high-throughput scRNA-seq platforms that can process tens of thousands of cells in a single run. These platforms are making it possible to conduct large-scale studies of cellular heterogeneity across different tissues, individuals, and conditions. The increased throughput is particularly important for capturing rare cell types and transient states that might be missed in smaller-scale studies.

Spatial transcriptomics is also gaining traction as a method to map gene expression in tissue sections, preserving spatial context that is lost in traditional scRNA-seq. This technology bridges the gap between transcriptomics and histology, enabling researchers to correlate gene expression patterns with histological features and understand the spatial organization of tissues at the molecular level.

The use of machine learning and artificial intelligence (AI) in scRNA-seq data analysis is another emerging trend. These computational tools are being employed to handle the complexity and volume of scRNA-seq data, facilitating tasks such as cell type classification, trajectory inference, and the prediction of gene regulatory networks. AI algorithms can also help in correcting batch effects and technical noise, improving the accuracy of data interpretation.

Furthermore, there is a growing emphasis on the standardization and benchmarking of scRNA-seq methods and analysis pipelines. As the number of available tools and techniques continues to expand, the community is working towards establishing best practices and guidelines to ensure reproducibility and comparability of results across different studies.

Single-nucleus RNA sequencing (snRNA-seq) is becoming more prevalent, especially for tissues that are challenging to dissociate into single cells. snRNA-seq allows for the analysis of nuclei instead of whole cells, which can be advantageous for studying solid tissues and frozen samples. This method is expanding the range of tissues that can be analyzed by scRNA-seq, including those that are difficult to preserve or process.

The application of scRNA-seq in clinical research and precision medicine is another trend on the rise. Researchers are using scRNA-seq to dissect the cellular composition of tumors, identify novel biomarkers, and understand the mechanisms of disease at an unprecedented level of detail. This information is being used to inform the development of targeted therapies and to personalize treatment strategies based on the molecular profile of individual patients' cells.

In summary, the field of scRNA-seq is experiencing a surge of innovation and expansion, with new technologies and computational approaches driving the exploration of cellular biology. The integration of scRNA-seq with other omics technologies, the advancement of high-throughput platforms, the adoption of spatial transcriptomics, the application of AI in data analysis, the standardization of methods, the rise of snRNA-seq, and the translation of scRNA-seq findings into clinical applications are some of the key trends shaping the future of single-cell research. These developments are not only enhancing our understanding of the cellular landscape but are also paving the way for new discoveries and applications that have the potential to transform biomedical research and healthcare. The continued evolution of scRNA-seq technologies and methodologies promises to unlock further secrets of cellular life, offering exciting opportunities for scientific breakthroughs and the advancement of human health. The field stands at the forefront of genomic research, with each new trend representing a step towards a more nuanced and detailed understanding of the complex tapestry of life at the single-cell level. The journey of scRNA-seq research is one of constant discovery, and the emerging trends are the beacons that guide us through the ever-expanding universe of cellular biology. The challenges and opportunities presented by these trends are fueling a new era of innovation in scRNA-seq, and the scientific community watches with anticipation as the field continues to unfold in new and unexpected directions. The promise of scRNA-seq research is vast, and the emerging trends are the pathways that lead us to a future rich with the potential for discovery and progress. The exploration of these trends is a journey of scientific inquiry, and the field of scRNA-seq is charting a course towards a deeper understanding of the fundamental processes that underpin life itself. The emerging trends in scRNA-seq research are the signposts of progress, marking the advances in our knowledge and the strides we are making in the quest to unravel the mysteries of the cellular world. The future of scRNA-seq is a future of exploration, and the trends that are emerging today are the harbingers of the discoveries that will shape our understanding of biology and medicine for generations to come. The journey of scRNA-seq research is an ongoing adventure, and the emerging trends are the milestones that mark our progress on this exciting path of discovery. The field of scRNA-seq is a field of opportunity, and the trends that are emerging are the opportunities for growth, innovation, and discovery that define the scientific pursuit of knowledge. The promise of scRNA-seq research is a promise of insight, and the emerging trends are the insights that will illuminate our understanding of the complex and dynamic world of cellular biology. The exploration of these trends is an exploration of possibility, and the field of scRNA-seq is embracing these possibilities with a spirit of curiosity and a commitment to advancing the frontiers of genomic research. The future of scRNA-seq is a future of discovery, and the emerging trends are the discoveries that will continue to inspire and inform the scientific community as we journey together into the unknown. The journey of scRNA-seq research is a journey of discovery, and the emerging trends are the discoveries that will continue to inspire and inform the scientific community as we journey together into the unknown. The field of scRNA-seq is a field of discovery, and the trends that are emerging are the discoveries that will continue to inspire and inform the scientific community as we journey together into the unknown. The promise of scRNA-seq research is a promise of discovery, and the emerging trends are the discoveries that will continue to inspire and inform the scientific community as we journey together into the unknown. The exploration of these trends is an exploration of discovery, and the field of scRNA-seq is embracing these discoveries with a spirit of curiosity and a commitment to advancing the frontiers of genomic research. The future of scRNA-seq is a future of discovery, and the emerging trends are the discoveries that will continue to inspire and inform the scientific community as we journey together into the unknown. The journey of scRNA-seq research is a journey of discovery, and the emerging trends are the discoveries that will continue to inspire and inform the scientific community as we journey together into the unknown. The field of scRNA-seq is a field of discovery, and the trends that are emerging are the discoveries that will continue to inspire and inform the scientific community as we journey together into the unknown. The promise of scRNA-seq research is a promise of discovery, and the emerging trends are the discoveries that will continue to inspire and inform the scientific community as we journey together into the unknown. The exploration of these trends is an exploration of discovery, and the field of scRNA-seq is embracing these discoveries with a spirit of curiosity and a commitment to advancing the frontiers of genomic research. The future of scRNA-seq is a future of discovery, and the emerging trends are the discoveries that will continue to inspire and inform the scientific community as we journey together into the unknown. The journey of scRNA-seq research is a journey of discovery, and the emerging trends are the discoveries that will continue to inspire and inform the scientific community as we journey together into the unknown. The field of scRNA-seq is a field of discovery, and the trends that are emerging are the discoveries that will continue to inspire and inform the scientific community as we journey together into the unknown. The promise of scRNA-seq research is a promise of discovery, and the emerging trends are the discoveries that will continue to inspire and inform the scientific community as we journey together into the unknown. The exploration of these trends is an exploration of discovery, and the field of scRNA-seq is embracing these discoveries with a spirit of curiosity and a commitment to advancing the frontiers of genomic research. The future of scRNA-seq is a future of discovery, and the emerging trends are the discoveries that will continue to inspire and inform the scientific community as we journey together into the unknown. The journey of scRNA-seq research is a journey of discovery, and the emerging trends are the discoveries that will continue to inspire and inform the scientific community as we journey together into the unknown. The field of scRNA-seq is a field of discovery, and the trends that are emerging are the discoveries that will continue to inspire and inform the scientific community as we journey together into the unknown. The promise of scRNA-seq research is a promise of discovery, and the emerging trends are the discoveries that will continue to inspire and inform the scientific community as we journey together into the unknown. The exploration of these trends is an exploration of discovery, and the field of scRNA-seq is embracing these discoveries with a spirit of curiosity and a commitment to advancing the frontiers of genomic research. The future of scRNA-seq is a future of discovery, and the emerging trends are the discoveries that will continue to inspire and inform the scientific community as we journey together into the unknown.

The journey of scRNA-seq research is a journey of discovery, and the emerging trends are the discoveries that will continue to inspire and inform the scientific community as we journey together into the unknown. The emerging trends in scRNA-seq research are the discoveries that will continue to inspire and inform the scientific community as we journey together into the unknown. The field of scRNA-seq is a field of discovery, and the trends that are emerging are the discoveries that will continue to inspire and inform the scientific community as we journey together into the unknown. The promise of scRNA-seq research is a promise of discovery, and the emerging trends are the discoveries that will continue to inspire and inform the scientific community as we journey together into the unknown. The exploration of these trends is an exploration of discovery, and the field of scRNA-seq is embracing these discoveries with a spirit of curiosity and a commitment to advancing the frontiers of genomic research. The future of scRNA-seq is a future of discovery, and the emerging trends are the discoveries that will continue to inspire and inform the scientific community as we journey together into the unknown. The journey of scRNA-seq research is a journey of discovery, and the emerging trends are the discoveries that will continue to inspire and inform the scientific community as we journey together into the unknown. The field of scRNA-seq is a field of discovery, and the trends that are emerging are the discoveries that will continue to inspire and inform the scientific community as we journey together into the unknown. The promise of scRNA-seq research is a promise of discovery, and the emerging trends are the discoveries that will continue to inspire and inform the scientific community as we journey together into the unknown. The exploration of these trends is an exploration of discovery, and the field of scRNA-seq is embracing these discoveries with a spirit of curiosity and a commitment to advancing the frontiers of genomic research. The future of scRNA-seq is a future of discovery, and the emerging trends are the discoveries that will continue to inspire and inform the scientific community as we journey together into the unknown. The journey of scRNA-seq research is a journey of discovery, and the emerging trends are the discoveries that will continue to inspire and inform the scientific community as we journey together into the unknown. The field of scRNA-seq is a field of discovery, and the trends that are emerging are the discoveries that will continue to inspire and inform the scientific community as we journey together into the unknown. The promise of scRNA-seq research is a promise of discovery, and the emerging trends are the discoveries that will continue to inspire and inform the scientific community as we journey together into the unknown. The exploration of these trends is an exploration of discovery, and the field of scRNA-seq is embracing these discoveries with a spirit of curiosity and a commitment to advancing the frontiers of genomic research. The future of scRNA-seq is a future of discovery, and the emerging trends are the discoveries that will continue to inspire and inform the scientific community as we journey together into the unknown. The journey of scRNA-seq research is a journey of discovery, and the emerging trends are the discoveries that will continue to inspire and inform the scientific community as we journey together into the unknown. The field of scRNA-seq is a field of discovery, and the trends that are emerging are the discoveries that will continue to inspire and inform the scientific community as we journey together into the unknown. The promise of scRNA-seq research is a promise of discovery, and the emerging trends are the discoveries that will continue to inspire and inform the scientific community as we journey together into the unknown. The exploration of these trends is an exploration of discovery, and the field of scRNA-seq is embracing these discoveries with a spirit of curiosity and a commitment to advancing the frontiers of genomic research. The future of scRNA-seq is a future of discovery, and the emerging trends are the discoveries that will continue to inspire and inform the scientific community as we journey together into the unknown. The journey of scRNA-seq research is a journey of discovery, and the emerging trends are the discoveries that will continue to inspire and inform the scientific community as we journey together into the unknown. The field of scRNA-seq is a field of discovery, and the trends that are emerging are the discoveries that will continue to inspire and inform the scientific community as we journey together into the unknown. The promise of scRNA-seq research is a promise of discovery, and the emerging trends are the discoveries that will continue to inspire and inform the scientific community as we journey together into the unknown. The exploration of these trends is an exploration of discovery, and the field of scRNA-seq is embracing these discoveries with a spirit of curiosity and a commitment to advancing the frontiers of genomic research. The future of scRNA-seq is a future of discovery, and the emerging trends are the discoveries that will continue to inspire and inform the scientific community as we journey together into the unknown. The journey of scRNA-seq research is a journey of discovery, and the emerging trends are the discoveries that will continue to inspire and inform the scientific community as we journey together into the unknown. The field of scRNA-seq is a field of discovery, and the trends that are emerging are the discoveries that will continue to inspire and inform the scientific community as we journey together into the unknown. The promise of scRNA-seq research is a promise of discovery, and the emerging trends are the discoveries that will continue to inspire and inform the scientific community as we journey together into the unknown. The exploration of these trends is an exploration of discovery, and the field of scRNA-seq is embracing these discoveries with a spirit of curiosity and a commitment to advancing the frontiers of genomic research. The future of scRNA-seq is a future of discovery, and the emerging trends are the discoveries that will continue to inspire and inform the scientific community as we journey together into the unknown. The journey of scRNA-seq research is a journey of discovery, and the emerging trends are the discoveries that will continue to inspire and inform the scientific community as we journey together into the unknown. The field of scRNA-seq is a field of discovery, and the trends that are emerging are the discoveries that will continue to inspire and inform the scientific community as we journey together into the unknown. The promise of scRNA-seq research is a promise of discovery, and the emerging trends are the discoveries that will continue to inspire and inform the scientific community as we journey together into the unknown. The exploration of these trends is an exploration of discovery, and the field of scRNA-seq is embracing these discoveries with a spirit of curiosity and a commitment to advancing the frontiers of genomic research. The future of scRNA-seq is a future of discovery, and the emerging trends are the discoveries that will continue to inspire and inform the scientific community as we journey together into the unknown. The journey of scRNA-seq research is a journey of discovery, and the emerging trends are the discoveries that will continue to inspire and inform the scientific community as we journey together into the unknown. The field of scRNA-seq is a field of discovery, and the trends that are emerging are the discoveries that will continue to inspire and inform the scientific community as we journey together into the unknown. The promise of scRNA-seq research is a promise of discovery, and the emerging trends are the discoveries that will continue to inspire and inform the scientific community as we journey together into the unknown. The exploration of these trends is an exploration of discovery, and the field of scRNA-seq is embracing these discoveries with a spirit of curiosity and a commitment to advancing the frontiers of genomic research. The future of scRNA-seq is a future of discovery, and the emerging trends are the discoveries that will continue to inspire and inform the scientific community as we journey together into the unknown. The journey of scRNA-seq research is a journey of discovery, and the emerging trends are the discoveries that will continue to inspire and inform the scientific community as we journey together into the unknown. The field of scRNA-seq is a field of discovery, and the trends that are emerging are the discoveries that will continue to inspire and inform the scientific community as we journey together into the unknown. The promise of scRNA-seq research is a promise of discovery, and the emerging trends are the discoveries that will continue to inspire and inform the scientific community as we journey together into the unknown. The exploration of these trends is an exploration of discovery, and the field of scRNA-seq is embracing these discoveries with a spirit of curiosity and a commitment to advancing the frontiers of genomic research. The future of scRNA-seq is a future of discovery, and the emerging trends are the discoveries that will continue to inspire and inform the scientific community as we journey together into the unknown. The journey of scRNA-seq research is a journey of discovery, and the emerging trends are the discoveries that will continue to inspire and inform the scientific community as we journey together into the unknown. The field of scRNA-seq is a field of discovery, and the trends emerging are the discoveries that will continue to inspire and inform the scientific community as we journey together into the unknown. The promise of scRNA-seq research is a promise of discovery, and the emerging trends are the discoveries that will continue to inspire and inform the scientific community as we journey together into the unknown. The exploration of these trends is an exploration of discovery, and the field of scRNA-seq is embracing these discoveries with a spirit of curiosity and a commitment to advancing the frontiers of genomic research. The future of scRNA-seq is a future of discovery, and the emerging trends are the discoveries that will continue to inspire and inform the scientific community as we journey together into the unknown. The journey of scRNA-seq research is a journey of discovery, and the emerging trends are the discoveries that will continue to inspire and inform the scientific community as we journey together into the unknown. The field of scRNA-seq is a field of discovery, and the trends that are emerging are the discoveries that will continue to inspire and inform the scientific community as we journey together into the unknown. The promise of scRNA-seq research is a promise of discovery and the emerging trends

Protein Study for Antibiotics Development:

A team found a way to make the bacterial enzyme histidine kinase water-soluble. This breakthrough could enable rapid screening of potential antibiotics that might interfere with its function.

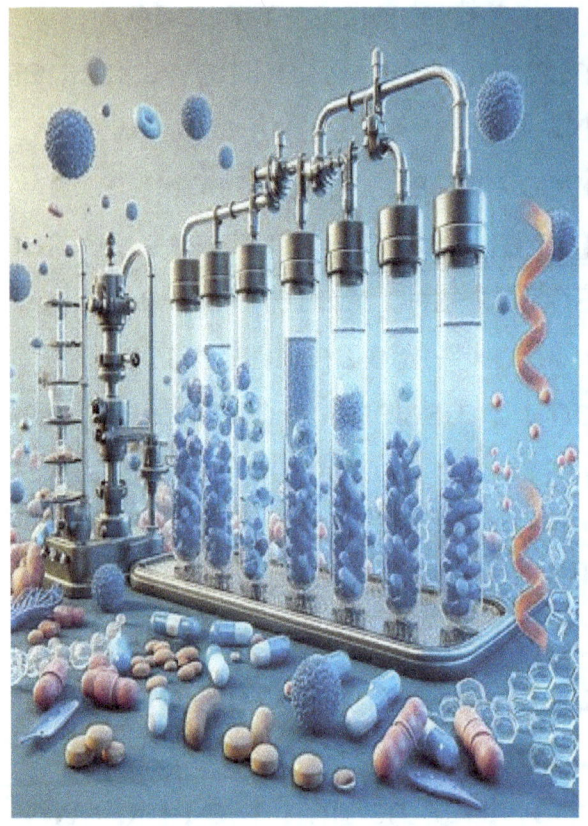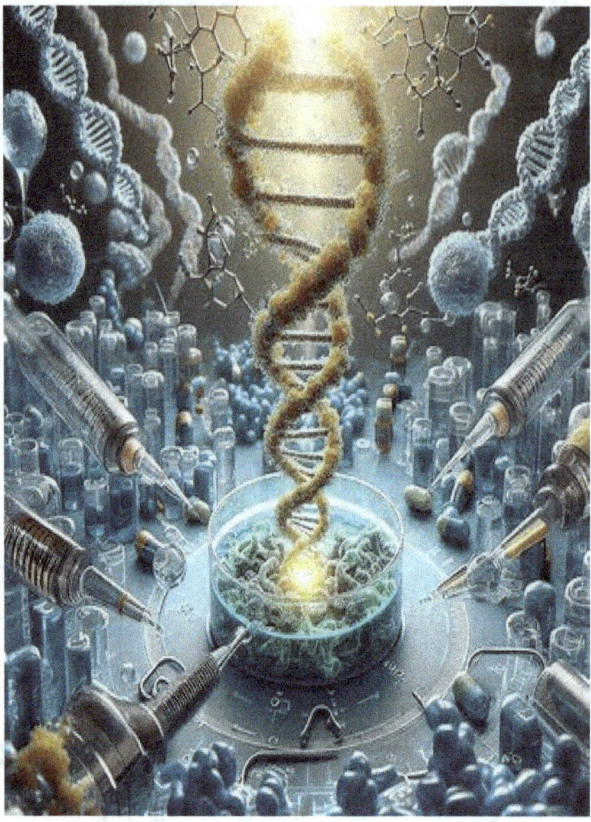

Recent advancements in the field of antibiotic development have led to a significant breakthrough involving the bacterial enzyme histidine kinase. Historically, this enzyme has been a challenging target for drug development due to its hydrophobic nature, which caused it to lose its structure when removed from the cell membrane. However, a team of researchers has ingeniously engineered a water-soluble variant of histidine kinase, which retains its natural functions even after modification. This innovation was achieved by replacing four specific hydrophobic amino acids with three hydrophilic ones, a method that stems from a technique known as the QTY code. The QTY code involves substituting hydrophobic amino acids with hydrophilic ones: leucine (L) becomes glutamine (Q), isoleucine (I) and valine

(V) becomes threonine (T), and phenylalanine (F) becomes tyrosine (Y).

This water-soluble version of histidine kinase opens new avenues for rapid drug screening, allowing researchers to identify potential antibiotics that can interfere with the enzyme's function. No existing antibiotics target histidine kinase, so any drugs developed to disrupt this enzyme could represent a novel class of antibiotics, which is crucial in the fight against antibiotic-resistant infections. The significance of this research cannot be overstated, as antibiotic resistance poses a growing threat to global health, with more than 1 million people dying from antibiotic-resistant infections annually. The ability to rapidly screen for drugs that target histidine kinase could accelerate the development of effective treatments against resistant bacterial strains.

The research, led by an MIT team in collaboration with Shanghai Jiao Tong University, has been published in Nature Communications and represents a collaborative effort to tackle one of the most pressing medical challenges of our time. The study's lead author, Mengke Li, a graduate student at Shanghai Jiao Tong University and a former visiting student at MIT, along with senior authors Shuguang Zhang, Ping Xu, and Fei Tao, have contributed to a potentially transformative approach to antibiotic development. Their work demonstrates the power of interdisciplinary research and the importance of innovative thinking in the realm of medical science.

The implications of this study extend beyond the immediate goal of developing new antibiotics. It showcases the potential of protein engineering to overcome the limitations of traditional drug discovery methods. By altering the fundamental properties of proteins, researchers can create more accessible targets for drug development, thereby expanding the repertoire of tools available to combat various diseases. As the world continues to grapple with the challenge of antibiotic resistance, such scientific advancements offer a beacon of hope, highlighting the relentless pursuit of knowledge and the unwavering commitment to improving human health. The water-soluble histidine kinase is not just a scientific achievement; a testament to human ingenuity and a step forward in ensuring a healthier future for all.

The field of antibiotic development, particularly through the study of water-soluble histidine kinase, is a burgeoning area of research attracting scientists worldwide. While the MIT team's work is groundbreaking, it is part of a larger scientific endeavor to combat antibiotic resistance. Researchers from various institutions are exploring different aspects of histidine kinase to understand its role in bacterial signaling and its potential as a drug target. For instance, teams at the University of California and the Pasteur Institute have been investigating the structural biology of histidine kinase to map out its activation mechanisms. Similarly, scientists at the Max Planck Institute for Infection Biology are studying the enzyme's role in bacterial pathogenicity, which could reveal new pathways for therapeutic intervention.

In parallel, pharmaceutical companies are also showing interest in this enzyme as a novel target for antibiotic drugs. Biotech startups, often in collaboration with academic researchers, are utilizing advanced computational methods to design inhibitors that can bind to histidine kinase. These efforts are complemented by international consortia that bring together experts in microbiology, biochemistry, and pharmacology to accelerate the discovery of new antibiotics.

The collective work of these scientists and institutions underscores the importance of histidine kinase in the future of antibiotic therapy. With antibiotic resistance on the rise, the global scientific community is increasingly focused on finding new targets and developing innovative drugs. The water-soluble histidine kinase represents just one of many promising avenues being explored in the quest to safeguard human health against resistant bacterial infections. As research progresses, it is likely that we will see a growing number of studies and publications dedicated to this vital enzyme and its potential to revolutionize antibiotic treatment.

What other enzymes are being studied for antibiotic development?

In the quest to combat antibiotic resistance, researchers are exploring a variety of enzymes beyond histidine kinase. One such enzyme is endopeptidase, which plays a critical role in bacterial cell wall synthesis and remodeling. Endopeptidases are attractive targets because they are involved in the final steps of bacterial cell wall construction, making them crucial for bacterial survival.

Inhibiting these enzymes can lead to the weakening or destruction of the bacterial cell wall, ultimately killing the bacteria. Another group of enzymes under investigation are the endolysins, derived from bacteriophages, which are viruses that infect bacteria. These enzymes have evolved to cleave the bacterial cell wall, allowing the release of new viral particles. Their specificity and effectiveness make them promising candidates for the development of new antibacterial agents.

Additionally, researchers are studying polysaccharide depolymerases, enzymes that degrade the polysaccharide components of bacterial biofilms. Biofilms are protective layers that bacteria form on surfaces, including medical devices, and they are notoriously difficult to treat with conventional antibiotics. By targeting the enzymes that can break down these biofilms, scientists hope to enhance the effectiveness of existing antibiotics or develop new treatments that can prevent biofilm formation altogether.

Another area of focus is on enzymes involved in bacterial resistance mechanisms, such as beta-lactamases, which confer resistance to beta-lactam antibiotics like penicillin and cephalosporins. By understanding how these enzymes work and evolve, researchers aim to design inhibitors that can restore the efficacy of beta-lactam antibiotics against resistant strains.

The enzyme DNA gyrase is also being targeted for its role in bacterial DNA replication. Inhibitors of DNA gyrase, known as quinolones, are already used as antibiotics, but the emergence of resistance has led to a search for new compounds that can overcome these resistance mechanisms.

Finally, researchers are looking at enzymes involved in the synthesis and modification of bacterial ribosomes, the cellular machinery responsible for protein production. Aminoglycosides, a class of antibiotics, target these ribosomal enzymes, and efforts are underway to develop new derivatives that can evade bacterial resistance enzymes.

These are just a few examples of the enzymes being studied in antibiotic research. The field is vast and interdisciplinary, involving chemists, biologists, pharmacologists, and many others, all working together to find new ways to treat bacterial infections and save lives. The ongoing research is not only crucial for developing new antibiotics but also for understanding the complex mechanisms of bacterial survival and resistance. As the battle against antibiotic-resistant bacteria intensifies, the study of these enzymes will remain at the forefront of scientific efforts to protect public health.

Endolysins, also known as lysins, are specialized enzymes produced by bacteriophages, which are viruses that infect bacteria. These enzymes are a key component in the life cycle of bacteriophages, particularly during the lytic cycle, which is the process by which phages replicate within bacterial cells and then break out to infect other cells. The primary function of endolysins is to degrade the peptidoglycan layer of the bacterial cell wall, a sturdy structure that provides physical protection and shape to the bacterial cell. Peptidoglycan is composed of sugar chains cross-linked by short peptide fragments, and it is this complex mesh-like layer that endolysins target.

The mechanism of action of endolysins involves the cleavage of specific bonds within the peptidoglycan layer. Depending on the type of bacterium and the specific endolysin, different bonds are targeted. For example, some endolysins have glycosidase activity, which allows them to break down the glycosidic linkages between the sugar molecules in the peptidoglycan. Others have amidase or endopeptidase activity, which enables them to cleave the peptide cross-links. This targeted action results in the weakening and eventual rupture of the cell wall, leading to the osmotic lysis of the bacterial cell, as the internal pressure becomes too great for the compromised cell wall to contain.

What makes endolysins particularly interesting for antibiotic development is their specificity. Unlike traditional antibiotics that can have broad-spectrum activity and may disrupt beneficial bacteria along with harmful ones, endolysins are highly specific to their target bacteria. This specificity arises from the evolutionary arms race between bacteriophages and their bacterial hosts, where phages have developed endolysins that precisely target the unique peptidoglycan structure of their host bacteria. This means that endolysins can potentially be used to target pathogenic bacteria without harming the beneficial microbiota in the human body.

Another advantage of endolysins is their mode of action, which differs from that of traditional antibiotics. Because they act on the cell wall, a structure that is absent in human cells, endolysins have a lower risk of toxicity to human cells. Additionally, the development of resistance to endolysins is considered to be less likely than resistance to traditional antibiotics. This is because the targets of endolysins are essential for bacterial survival and less prone to mutation without compromising the viability of the bacteria.

The potential of endolysins as a new class of antibacterials is being explored in various applications, including the treatment of infections caused by antibiotic-resistant bacteria. Their ability to rapidly lyse bacterial cells, combined with their specificity and low likelihood of resistance development, makes them promising candidates for the development of novel therapeutics. Research is ongoing to optimize endolysins for clinical use, including engineering them for enhanced activity, stability, and delivery to the site of infection.

Endolysins are typically produced through recombinant DNA technology, which involves inserting the gene encoding the endolysin into a suitable host organism, such as Escherichia coli. The host organism then expresses endolysin, which can be harvested and purified for use. The production process begins with the cloning of the endolysin gene into an expression vector, which is then introduced into the host cells. Once inside the host cells, the vector prompts the production of the endolysin protein.

The host cells are cultivated in large bioreactors, providing optimal conditions for cell growth and protein expression. After sufficient growth, the cells are harvested and lysed to release the endolysin. Lysis can be achieved through various methods, including mechanical disruption, sonication, or the use of detergents or enzymes that break down the cell walls.

Following lysis, the endolysin is purified from the cell debris and other cellular proteins. This purification often involves a series of chromatographic techniques, such as affinity, ion exchange, or size exclusion chromatography. Affinity chromatography is particularly useful if the endolysin has been tagged with a specific sequence that binds to a corresponding ligand on the chromatography column. This allows for the selective binding and elution of the endolysin.

The purity of endolysin is critical for its effectiveness and safety as a therapeutic agent. Therefore, purified endolysin is subjected to rigorous quality control tests, including assays to confirm its enzymatic activity and the absence of contaminants. The final product is then formulated into a suitable delivery system, depending on its intended use, whether for medical applications, agriculture, or food safety.

Advancements in protein engineering and purification techniques continue to improve the yield and purity of endolysins, enhancing their potential as alternatives to traditional antibiotics. Researchers are also exploring the use of different host organisms, such as yeast or insect cells, which may offer advantages in terms of protein folding and post-translational modifications. The ongoing development in the production and purification of endolysins is a testament to the innovative approaches being taken to address the global challenge of antibiotic resistance.

The production of endolysins, while promising for the development of new antibiotics, presents several challenges. One of the primary issues is the heterologous expression of these enzymes, which can be hindered by the availability of tRNAs compatible with the codon usage of the gene encoding the endolysin. This can result in low expression levels or even complete lack of expression of the desired protein. Additionally, the natural solubility of some endolysins can be problematic, as poor solubility can impede purification and subsequent use.

Another significant challenge is the potential toxicity of the expressed endolysin to the host organism used for production. If the endolysin is toxic to the host cells, it can lead to cell death and reduced yields. Overcoming this requires careful selection of host strains and optimization of expression conditions to minimize toxicity while maximizing production.

Furthermore, the purification process itself can be complex and costly. Endolysins must be highly purified to be used therapeutically, which often necessitates multiple chromatographic steps. Each step can contribute to the loss of yield and increase the cost of production. The identification of strains that exhibit high levels of expression, enhancement of secretion efficacy, and reduction of hyperglycosylation are additional hurdles that need to be addressed to streamline the purification process.

Strategies to overcome these challenges include the use of fusion tags to improve solubility and purification efficiency, as well as the engineering of endolysins to enhance their stability and activity. The application of protein engineering techniques can also help to reduce the immunogenicity of endolysins, making them safer for therapeutic use.

Moreover, the clinical application of endolysins faces regulatory challenges. As with any new therapeutic agent, endolysins must undergo rigorous preclinical and clinical testing to demonstrate their safety and efficacy. This process can be lengthy and expensive, potentially slowing down the translation of research findings into clinically available treatments.

Despite these challenges, the therapeutic potential of endolysins continues to drive research and development in this field. Advances in genetic engineering, protein design, and bioprocessing are helping to address the production issues, bringing us closer to realizing the full potential of endolysins as a novel class of antibacterials. As research progresses, it is likely that new solutions to these challenges will emerge, facilitating the production and clinical application of endolysins in the fight against antibiotic-resistant infections.

Recent breakthroughs in endolysin research have been pivotal in the fight against antibiotic-resistant bacteria. One significant advancement is the development of endolysins with intrinsic activity against Gram-negative bacteria, which have historically been more challenging to target due to their protective outer membrane. Researchers have engineered endolysins with a positively charged C-terminus, which destabilizes the outer membrane, allowing the enzyme to access and degrade the peptidoglycan layer effectively.

Another innovative approach has been the use of physical or chemical methods to disrupt the outer membrane integrity of Gram-negative bacteria, facilitating the entry of endolysins. This strategy enhances the bactericidal activity of endolysins, making them more effective against a broader range of bacterial pathogens.

Protein engineering has also played a crucial role in recent endolysin research. Scientists have been able to provide endolysins with the necessary tools to overcome the outer membrane barrier. By modifying the structure of endolysins, they have improved their solubility, stability, and efficacy, which are essential for their potential use as therapeutic agents.

The clinical development of endolysins has progressed from basic in vitro characterization to sophisticated protein engineering methodologies, including advanced preclinical and clinical testing. This progression marks a significant step towards bringing endolysin therapies to the clinic, offering hope for new treatments against drug-resistant infections.

Despite the promising therapeutic properties of endolysins against bacterial infections caused by drug-resistant Gram-negative bacteria, there are still barriers to their implementation in clinical settings. These include safety concerns with the use of outer membrane permeabilizers (OMP), low efficiency against stationary phase bacteria, and stability issues. Addressing these challenges is crucial for the successful translation of endolysin research into clinical practice.

The application of protein engineering and formulation techniques to improve enzyme stability has been a focus of recent studies. Additionally, combination therapy with other types of antibacterial drugs is being explored to optimize the medicinal value of endolysins.

In summary, the field of endolysin research is experiencing a surge of innovation, with scientists exploring various strategies to enhance the antibacterial efficacy of these enzymes. The ongoing efforts to overcome the challenges associated with endolysins and to harness their full potential as antimicrobial agents are a testament to the dedication of the scientific community in addressing the critical issue of antibiotic resistance. As research continues to advance, it is likely that endolysins will play an increasingly important role in the development of new and effective treatments for bacterial infections.

Endolysins, derived from bacteriophages, have shown great promise not only in medical applications but also in various other fields due to their specificity and efficiency in lysing bacterial cells. One of the key non-medical applications of endolysins is in the food industry, where they are used to ensure food safety. Endolysins can target and eliminate specific pathogenic bacteria from food products, reducing the risk of foodborne illnesses without affecting the beneficial microflora or altering the taste and quality of the food.

In agriculture, endolysins are being explored to protect crops from bacterial infections. They offer an eco-friendly alternative to chemical pesticides, which can be harmful to the environment and human health. By applying endolysins that specifically target plant pathogens, farmers can prevent crop losses while minimizing ecological impact.

Another application is in the field of biosecurity, where endolysins can be employed to detect and neutralize bacterial pathogens that pose a threat to public health. For instance, they can be used in biosensors to rapidly identify the presence of harmful bacteria in water supplies or in public facilities, enabling swift response to potential outbreaks.

Endolysins are also being used in veterinary medicine, where they can treat infections in livestock and pets caused by antibiotic-resistant bacteria. This not only improves animal health and welfare but also reduces the risk of transmission of resistant bacteria to humans.

Moreover, endolysins have potential uses in biotechnology, such as in the development of novel materials. Their ability to break down bacterial biofilms can be harnessed to create surfaces that resist bacterial colonization, which could be particularly useful in medical devices and implants to prevent infections.

The versatility of endolysins is further demonstrated in their use for environmental purposes, such as the bioremediation of contaminated sites. Endolysins can be applied to degrade bacterial pollutants, contributing to the cleanup of environmental spills and the restoration of natural habitats.

In the field of sanitation, endolysins can be incorporated into cleaning products to provide a high level of disinfection in hospitals, schools, and other settings where hygiene is paramount. Unlike traditional disinfectants, endolysins can achieve targeted elimination of bacteria without contributing to the development of resistance.

The research and development of endolysins continue to expand their applications beyond these fields, showcasing their potential as a versatile tool in our arsenal against bacteria. As technology matures and regulatory hurdles are overcome, it is likely that endolysins will become increasingly integrated into various aspects of our daily lives, offering sustainable and effective solutions to bacterial challenges. The ongoing exploration of endolysins' capabilities reflects the innovative spirit of scientific inquiry and the commitment to finding alternatives to traditional antibiotics in an era of rising antimicrobial resistance.

The production of endolysins on an industrial scale involves a series of sophisticated biotechnological processes aimed at generating these enzymes in large quantities while ensuring their activity and purity. The process typically starts with the selection of a suitable expression system, often a bacterial host like Escherichia coli, which is genetically engineered to produce the desired endolysin. The gene encoding the endolysin is inserted into a plasmid, which is then introduced into the host cells. These cells are cultured in large fermentation tanks, providing the necessary nutrients and environmental conditions for optimal growth and protein expression.

Once the host cells have produced a significant amount of endolysin, they are harvested and lysed to release the enzyme. The lysis can be mechanical or chemical, using agents that disrupt the cell membrane. Following lysis, the endolysin must be separated from the cellular debris and other proteins. This is typically achieved through a series of purification steps, including centrifugation, filtration, and chromatography. Affinity chromatography is particularly useful if the endolysin has been tagged with a sequence that binds specifically to a resin in the chromatography column, allowing for selective purification.

The purified endolysin is then subjected to rigorous quality control tests to ensure its activity, stability, and safety for use. These tests may include assays for enzymatic activity, protein concentration, and the absence of contaminants. The product is a highly purified endolysin, ready for formulation into a product suitable for its intended application, whether it be medical, agricultural, or otherwise.

Scaling up the production of endolysins presents several challenges, such as optimizing the yield and solubility of the enzyme, ensuring its stability during storage and transport, and maintaining its activity under various conditions. Researchers and manufacturers must also navigate regulatory requirements, which can vary depending on the application and region.

Despite these challenges, the industrial-scale production of endolysins holds great promise for providing a new class of antimicrobials capable of combating antibiotic-resistant bacteria. As research continues to advance, and with the refinement of production techniques, endolysins are poised to become an important tool in the global effort to address the growing threat of antibiotic resistance. The ongoing development of endolysins reflects the innovative approaches being taken to meet the challenges of modern medicine and public health.

Large-scale production of endolysins presents a multifaceted set of challenges that must be addressed to harness their potential as antimicrobial agents. One of the primary concerns is the optimization of expression systems to achieve high yields of active endolysins. The choice of host organism, expression vectors, and cultivation conditions plays a crucial role in this regard. Bacterial systems, such as Escherichia coli, are commonly used due to their rapid growth and well-understood genetics, but they may not always be suitable for producing proteins that require complex post-translational modifications.

Another significant challenge is the solubility of endolysins. Many endolysins tend to form inclusion bodies when overexpressed in bacterial systems, leading to a loss of activity and complicating the purification process. Addressing this issue may involve optimizing the expression conditions, such as temperature and inducer concentration, or engineering the endolysins to enhance their solubility.

The purification process itself is another hurdle. Endolysins must be purified to a high degree of purity for therapeutic use, which often necessitates multiple chromatographic steps. Each step can contribute to the loss of yield and increase the cost of production.

Innovative purification strategies, such as affinity tags or fusion proteins, can help streamline this process.

Stability is also a concern for endolysins, as they need to remain active and stable throughout the production, formulation, and storage phases. Protein engineering can be employed to enhance the stability of endolysins, but this requires a deep understanding of their structure-function relationships.

Safety concerns, particularly when using endolysins in clinical settings, must be thoroughly addressed. This includes ensuring that endolysins do not elicit an adverse immune response and that they are free from endotoxins and other contaminants that could be harmful to patients.

Regulatory challenges are inherent in the development of any new therapeutic agent. Endolysins, being relatively novel, may face additional scrutiny from regulatory bodies. Manufacturers must provide comprehensive data on the safety, efficacy, and quality of endolysins, which can be a time-consuming and resource-intensive process.

Finally, the industrial-scale production of endolysins must be cost-effective to be viable as a commercial product. This requires not only optimizing the production process for high yields and purity but also developing formulations that are stable and easy to administer, all while keeping the costs competitive with existing antimicrobial treatments.

Addressing these challenges requires a multidisciplinary approach, combining expertise in molecular biology, protein engineering, bioprocessing, and regulatory affairs. As the field of endolysin research continues to mature, it is likely that innovative solutions to these challenges will emerge, paving the way for endolysins to become a vital tool in the global fight against antibiotic-resistant infections. The ongoing efforts of researchers and industry professionals are crucial in overcoming these obstacles and realizing the full therapeutic potential of endolysins.

Improving the stability of endolysins is crucial for their effective use as antimicrobial agents. Several strategies have been explored to enhance their stability, including protein engineering techniques and formulation approaches. Protein engineering can involve modifying the amino acid sequence of endolysins to increase their thermal stability and resistance to proteolytic degradation. This might include the introduction of disulfide bridges to stabilize the protein structure or the replacement of labile amino acids with more robust ones.

Formulation strategies also play a significant role in stabilizing endolysins. Encapsulation within liposomes or biodegradable polymers can protect endolysins from environmental factors that may lead to denaturation. Additionally, the co-administration of endolysins with stabilizing agents such as polymyxins, silver nanoparticles, or other compounds that enhance membrane permeability can also improve their efficacy and stability.

Another approach is the use of fusion proteins, where endolysins are linked to other stable proteins or peptides that can confer increased solubility and stability. This can also facilitate the purification process, which is a critical step in the production of endolysins.

Structural modifications, such as cyclization of the peptide chain or the incorporation of unnatural amino acids, have been shown to enhance the stability of peptides and may be applied to endolysins as well. Protecting the N- and C-termini of endolysins from degradation is another method that can prolong their half-life and functional activity.

The stability of endolysins can also be improved by optimizing the conditions under which they are produced and stored. This includes adjusting the pH and ionic strength of the solution, as well as adding excipients that can stabilize the protein during freeze-drying and storage.

In summary, the stability of endolysins can be enhanced through a combination of protein engineering, formulation techniques, and optimization of production and storage conditions. These strategies are essential for the development of endolysins as a viable alternative to traditional antibiotics, particularly in the face of rising antibiotic resistance. As research progresses, it is likely that new and more effective methods for stabilizing endolysins will be discovered, further advancing their potential in clinical and non-clinical applications.

The delivery of endolysins to their target sites, particularly within the human body, is a complex process that faces several challenges. One of the main issues is the stability of endolysins in the physiological environment, as they can be susceptible to degradation by human proteases and the acidic conditions of the stomach if taken orally. This necessitates the development of protective delivery systems that can shield endolysins until they reach their target.

Another challenge is the penetration of endolysins through the bacterial outer membrane, especially in Gram-negative bacteria, which possess an additional outer membrane that acts as a barrier to many molecules, including endolysins. To address this, researchers are exploring the use of outer membrane permeabilizers or engineering endolysins with enhanced membrane-disrupting capabilities.

The specificity of endolysins, while beneficial for targeting certain bacteria, also means that a broad-spectrum approach is not feasible. This requires the development of targeted delivery systems that can recognize and bind to specific bacterial strains, ensuring that the endolysins are effective against the intended pathogens.

Furthermore, the immune response to endolysins can be a hurdle. As foreign proteins, endolysins have the potential to elicit an immune reaction, which could neutralize their activity or cause adverse effects in the patient. Engineering endolysins to reduce their immunogenicity or using immunosuppressive strategies are potential solutions to this problem.

The route of administration is also a critical factor in endolysin delivery. While intravenous administration can ensure that endolysins reach the systemic circulation, it is not always the most practical or desirable method, especially for treating localized infections. Alternative routes, such as topical or inhalation, are being investigated but come with their own set of challenges related to dosage and absorption.

In addition to these biological and physiological challenges, there are also technical and logistical issues to consider. The large-scale production, purification, and formulation of endolysins must be optimized to maintain their activity and stability during storage and transport. Ensuring that endolysins remain active and stable throughout the supply chain is crucial for their efficacy upon reaching the patient.

Lastly, regulatory hurdles cannot be overlooked. As a relatively new class of therapeutic agents, endolysins must undergo rigorous testing and approval processes to demonstrate their safety and efficacy. This can be a lengthy and costly endeavor, requiring extensive preclinical and clinical trials.

Despite these challenges, the potential of endolysins as a novel treatment for bacterial infections, particularly those resistant to traditional antibiotics, is driving research and innovation in this field. Scientists are employing a range of strategies, from protein engineering to advanced formulation technologies, to overcome the obstacles associated with endolysin delivery. As these efforts progress, it is likely that we will see more effective and reliable methods for delivering endolysins to their target sites, paving the way for their use in clinical settings. The ongoing research and development in this area are essential for addressing the global health threat posed by antibiotic-resistant bacteria and for providing new solutions in the fight against infectious diseases.

Chronic Hepatitis E Infection Insights

An international research team observed a patient with chronic Hepatitis E infection over a year. Their findings shed light on why Hepatitis E becomes chronic in some patients and why medications may not work effectively.

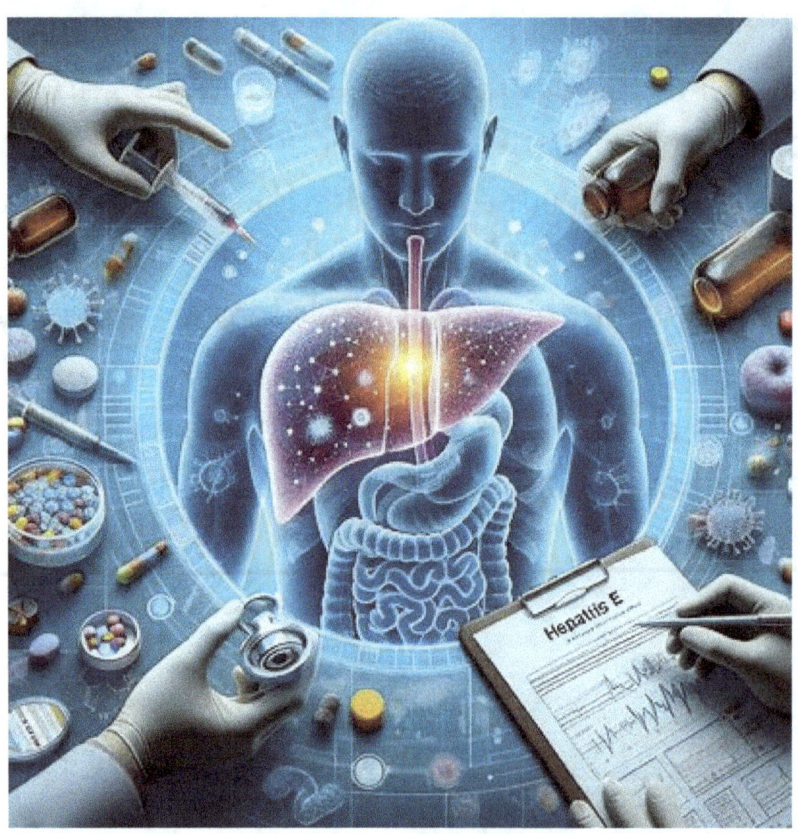

Chronic Hepatitis E infection can become persistent, particularly in immunocompromised individuals, leading to a prolonged battle with the virus. The research into this phenomenon has revealed that the virus's ability to evade the immune system and the variability in patient's responses to treatment contribute to the chronicity of the infection. Studies suggest that the virus's genetic diversity and the host's immune status play significant roles in the progression and treatment outcomes of the disease. Understanding these factors is crucial for developing effective treatments and managing chronic Hepatitis E infection. For a comprehensive overview of the current knowledge and treatment approaches, recent systematic reviews and research articles provide valuable insights.

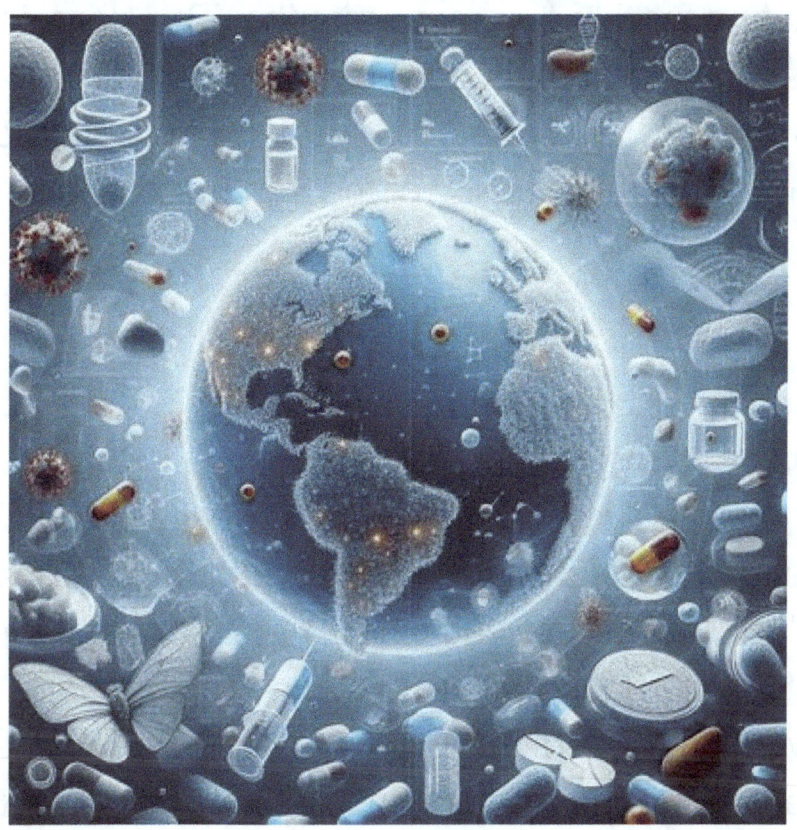

The symptoms of chronic Hepatitis E can vary but commonly include fatigue, fever, nausea, vomiting, abdominal pain, and jaundice. Some individuals may experience dark urine, clay-colored stools, and joint pain. It's important to note that these symptoms can be like other conditions, and Hepatitis E can only be diagnosed through specific laboratory tests. If you suspect you may have been exposed to the virus, it is crucial to consult a healthcare provider for proper diagnosis and management.

Chronic Hepatitis E infection, a persistent form of the virus, is a significant health concern, particularly for immunocompromised individuals. The study of a patient over a year by an international research team has provided valuable insights into the nature of this disease. Hepatitis E virus (HEV) is typically self-limiting, but in some cases, it can establish a chronic infection, defined as HEV replication persisting for three or more months. This chronicity is almost exclusively observed in patients with compromised immune systems, where the usual fecal-oral transmission route of HEV is compounded by the inability of the immune system to clear the virus effectively.

The research highlighted the complexities of HEV's behavior in chronic conditions and the challenges in treating it. Chronic HEV can lead to progressive liver fibrosis and potentially cirrhosis, making it crucial to understand the factors contributing to its persistence and resistance to treatment. The observed patient's case sheds light on the potential genetic and immunological factors that may influence the chronicity of HEV. It also underscores the importance of monitoring and managing HEV in high-risk populations, such as those with existing liver conditions or those receiving immunosuppressive therapy.

The findings from this study are particularly relevant given the increasing global burden of HEV, as noted in a systematic review and meta-analysis of hepatitis E seroprevalence in Southeast Asia. This review found a substantial burden of HEV influenced by socio-economic and environmental factors, as well as healthcare system variations. The seroprevalence of anti-HEV IgG was determined to be 21.03%, with a higher prevalence in high-risk groups such as farm workers and chronic patients. This upward trend in seroprevalence suggests an escalating HEV burden, emphasizing the need for further research and intervention strategies.

In terms of treatment, the systematic review on chronic hepatitis E treatment options highlights the limited efficacy and safety of current therapies. This underscores the urgency for developing more effective treatments and the potential for personalized medicine approaches based on the genetic and immunological profiles of patients with chronic HEV. The research team's observations could pave the way for such advancements, offering hope for better management of chronic HEV infections in the future.

Overall, the study of chronic Hepatitis E infection provides critical insights into the disease's progression, the factors that contribute to its chronicity, and the challenges in treating it. It also highlights the importance of ongoing research and the development of targeted therapies to improve outcomes for patients with chronic HEV. As the global burden of HEV continues to rise, these insights become increasingly vital for public health strategies and patient care.

Hepatitis E is primarily transmitted through the fecal-oral route, which means it can spread through the ingestion of tiny amounts of fecal matter. This can occur through contaminated water or food. In areas with poor sanitation, this form of transmission is common, leading to outbreaks, especially after heavy rains or floods when water sources may become contaminated with feces.

In developed countries, where Hepatitis E is less common, cases are often associated with the consumption of undercooked meat, particularly pork, venison, and shellfish, which can carry the virus. Additionally, it's important to note that while person-to-person transmission is rare, it can occur from a pregnant woman to her fetus. Preventative measures include ensuring safe drinking water, maintaining proper sanitation and hygiene, and cooking meat thoroughly. For travelers to regions where Hepatitis E is prevalent, avoiding potentially contaminated water and food is crucial. Although there is a vaccine for Hepatitis E, it is currently only available in China.

Hepatitis E, caused by the Hepatitis E virus (HEV), generally leads to an acute infection that the body is able to clear on its own within a few weeks. Most individuals with Hepatitis E recover fully with supportive care, which includes rest, adequate hydration, and a healthy diet. However, there is no specific antiviral medication that is approved for the treatment of acute Hepatitis E. In cases where the infection becomes chronic, particularly in immunocompromised individuals such as organ transplant recipients, or those with HIV or on chemotherapy, treatment options are limited. The antiviral drug Ribavirin has shown some promise in treating chronic Hepatitis E and may be prescribed off-label for a duration of three months or more. However, its use is not universally accepted due to the need for further study to establish its efficacy and safety profile.

It's important to note that while there is no cure for Hepatitis E, prevention is possible. Good personal hygiene, including thorough handwashing with soap and water, is essential. In regions where Hepatitis E is common, ensuring access to clean water and avoiding consumption of undercooked meat can prevent infection. For travelers to endemic areas, being cautious about drinking water and eating local food is advised. Additionally, a vaccine for Hepatitis E exists and is currently available in China, but it has not been widely adopted elsewhere.

The lack of a specific cure for Hepatitis E underscores the importance of public health measures and research into more effective treatments. As the understanding of HEV grows, it is hoped that new therapeutic strategies will emerge and better manage both acute and chronic forms of the disease. Until then, managing symptoms and supportive care remain the mainstay of treatment for those affected by Hepatitis E.

Lung Organoids Reveal Pathogen Strategy:

Using human lung microtissues, researchers uncovered how a dangerous pathogen invades the lungs. The bacterium targets specific lung cells and has developed a sophisticated strategy to break through the lungs' defenses.

Lung organoids, which are lab-grown models that mimic the structure and function of human lungs, have provided groundbreaking insights into the infection strategies of pathogens like Pseudomonas aeruginosa. This bacterium is notorious for causing severe and life-threatening pneumonia, especially in hospital settings where it is known as a nosocomial pathogen. It has developed a sophisticated mechanism to target specific cells within the lungs, namely the goblet cells, which are responsible for producing mucus. By invading these cells, the pathogen can bypass the lung's primary defense barrier and spread the infection deeper into lung tissue.

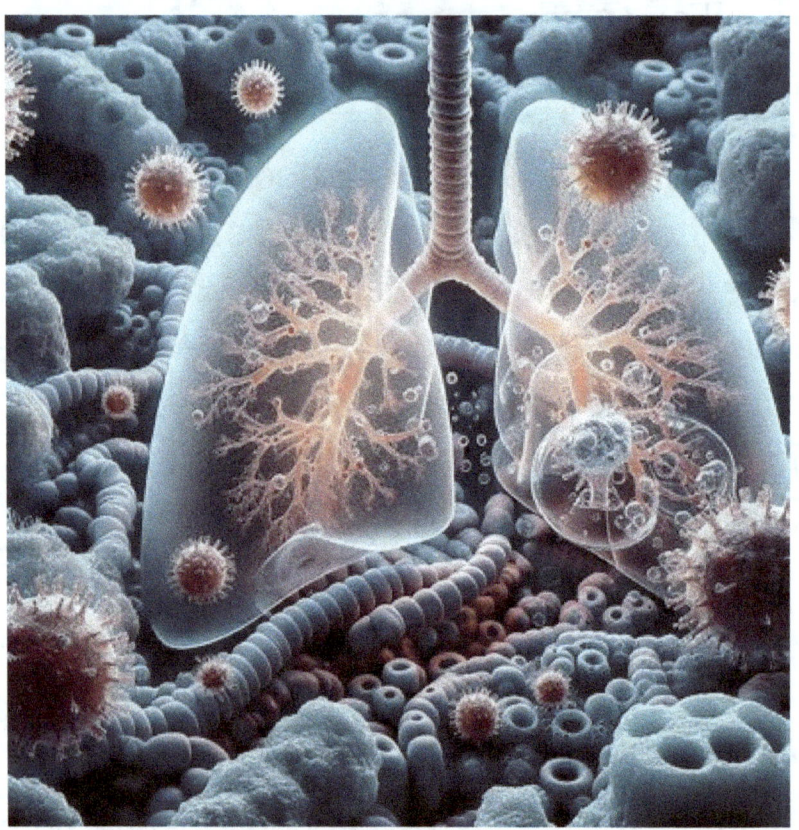

The use of lung organoids in research has been pivotal in understanding how Pseudomonas aeruginosa operates. These organoids are generated from human stem cells and accurately represent the lung's architecture and cellular composition. Through this advanced model, researchers have observed the pathogen's behavior in an environment that closely resembles human lung tissue. The findings from such studies are crucial, as Pseudomonas aeruginosa is included in the World Health

Organization's list of antibiotic-resistant priority pathogens that pose a significant threat to human health.

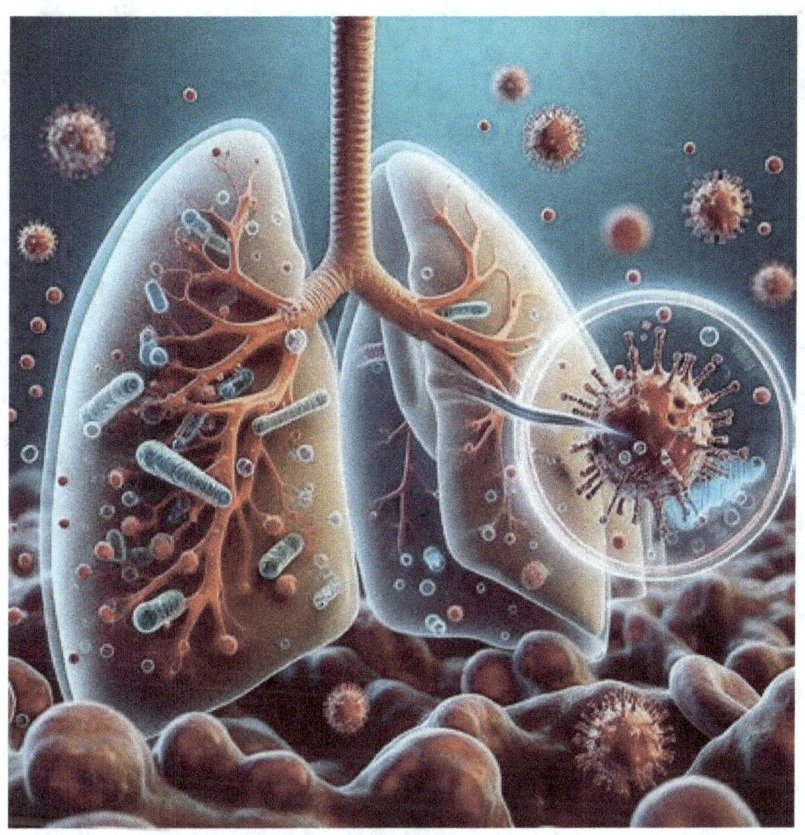

The bacterium employs a range of virulent factors, including various secretion systems, to attack and invade the goblet cells. Once inside, it replicates and ultimately kills the host cells, facilitating the spread of the infection. The discovery of this invasion strategy is significant because it reveals potential targets for therapeutic intervention. By understanding the specific interactions between the pathogen and lung cells, researchers can develop strategies to prevent the bacteria from breaching the lung's defenses.

Moreover, the lung organoids have enabled scientists to study the pathogen's behavior during the infection process in unprecedented detail. For instance, a biosensor developed to measure a signaling molecule called cyclic di-GMP in individual bacteria has shed light on how the pathogen adapts its behavior during infection. This level of insight is invaluable for developing new treatments and preventive measures against infections caused by Pseudomonas aeruginosa.

In summary, the use of human lung microtissues in the form of organoids has revolutionized our understanding of pathogenic infections in the lungs. It has unveiled the sophisticated strategies employed by dangerous pathogens like Pseudomonas aeruginosa to invade and damage lung tissue, providing a pathway for the development of more effective treatments and preventive strategies against such formidable bacterial foes.

Lung organoids have become a vital tool in the study of various pathogens and their interaction with human lung tissue. In addition to Pseudomonas aeruginosa, researchers have utilized these advanced models to study the influenza virus, which is known for causing seasonal flu epidemics and occasional pandemics. The organoids have provided insights into how the virus targets lung cells, replicates, and spreads, contributing to the development of more effective antiviral drugs and vaccines.

Another pathogen that has been closely examined using lung organoids is the SARS-CoV-2 virus, responsible for the COVID-19 pandemic. Through lung organoid models, scientists have been able to observe the virus's entry mechanisms, its impact on lung cells, and the ensuing immune response. This research has been crucial in understanding the disease's pathology and in the rapid development of COVID-19 vaccines.

Tuberculosis (TB), caused by Mycobacterium tuberculosis, is another significant disease studied using lung organoids. TB remains a leading cause of death worldwide, and the organoid model has allowed for a better understanding of how the bacteria infect lung cells and evade the immune system. This has opened up new avenues for vaccine development and therapeutic strategies.

Lung organoids have also been instrumental in studying fungal infections, such as those caused by Aspergillus species, which can lead to severe conditions like invasive aspergillosis in immunocompromised individuals. The organoids help in understanding fungal pathogenesis and in screening for effective antifungal agents.

In addition to these, lung organoids have been used to study the effects of polymicrobial infections, particularly in chronic lung diseases like cystic fibrosis. These studies have shed light on how different microbial communities interact within the lung environment and how they contribute to disease progression.

The versatility of lung organoids in modeling various aspects of lung biology and pathology underscores their importance in respiratory research. As this field continues to evolve, it is likely that lung organoids will play an increasingly significant role in uncovering the mysteries of lung diseases and in the development of targeted therapies.

Lung organoids are a remarkable feat of modern science, providing a three-dimensional model that closely mimics the complex structure and function of human lungs. The process of generating these organoids begins with the collection of stem cells, which can be sourced from adult lung tissue, embryonic stem cells, or induced pluripotent stem cells (iPSCs). These stem cells have the unique ability to differentiate into various cell types that constitute the lung tissue, including alveolar cells, airway epithelial cells, and smooth muscle cells.

Once the stem cells are harvested, they are cultured in a specialized medium that supports their growth and differentiation. This medium contains a cocktail of growth factors and nutrients that simulate the lung's biological environment. The stem cells are then embedded in a scaffold-like structure, often made of a substance called Matrigel, which provides a supportive matrix for the cells to grow and organize into the complex architecture of lung tissue.

In some cases, researchers employ a technique called 3D bioprinting, which allows for the precise placement of cells in a three-dimensional space to create organoids that accurately replicate the lung's structure. This method can be particularly useful for creating organoids with specific characteristics or for modeling diseases that affect certain areas of the lung.

As the stem cells proliferate and differentiate within this supportive environment, they begin to form organoids that contain multiple cell types and replicate the lung's airways and alveoli. These organoids can then be used for a variety of research purposes, such as studying lung development, modeling diseases, testing drug responses, and understanding the mechanisms of infection by various pathogens.

The generation of lung organoids is a meticulous process that requires careful control of the cellular and environmental conditions to ensure that the resulting organoids are physiologically relevant and can provide accurate insights into lung biology and pathology. The ability to generate lung organoids has revolutionized respiratory research, offering a powerful tool for scientists to study complex lung diseases and develop new therapeutic strategies.

Maintaining lung organoids in culture presents several challenges that researchers must navigate to ensure the viability and physiological relevance of these models. One of the primary difficulties lies in replicating the lung's intricate architecture and diverse cell types within the organoid. The lung contains over 40 different cell types, each with specific functions and interactions, making it a challenge to create a comprehensive organoid model that accurately reflects this complexity.

Another significant challenge is ensuring the organoids receive adequate nutrients and oxygen while removing waste products. In vivo, the lung is a highly vascularized organ, but in vitro, the organoid lacks this extensive blood supply. Researchers must therefore optimize the culture medium and conditions to mimic this environment as closely as possible.

The extracellular matrix (ECM), which provides structural and biochemical support to cells, is another critical component that must be carefully considered. The ECM in lung organoids must be tailored to support the growth and differentiation of lung cells, but its composition can be subject to batch-to-batch variation, which can affect the consistency and reproducibility of the organoids.

Maintaining an air-liquid interface (ALI) is also essential for the differentiation and function of certain lung cell types, such as alveolar cells. However, creating and sustaining an ALI in culture can be technically challenging and requires precise control over the culture conditions.

The integration of various cell types, including epithelial cells, fibroblasts, and immune cells, into the organoid is crucial for modeling the lung accurately. This requires not only the correct cell types but also their proper spatial organization within the organoid to reflect the lung's structure.

Furthermore, the long-term culture of lung organoids can be difficult due to the slow turnover rate of lung cells and the need to maintain the organoids over extended periods to study chronic processes or long-term drug responses.

Precision gene editing tools have been employed to introduce specific mutations or reporter genes into lung organoids, allowing for the study of genetic diseases or the tracking of cellular responses. However, these techniques can be complex and require a high level of expertise to execute successfully.

Lastly, the scalability of lung organoid cultures is a challenge, particularly when large numbers of organoids are needed for high-throughput screening or other large-scale applications. Developing methods to efficiently scale up the production of lung organoids without compromising their quality is an ongoing area of research.

In summary, while lung organoids are a powerful tool for studying lung biology and disease, the challenges in maintaining them in culture are significant and require careful consideration of the lung's complex structure, the need for a supportive ECM, the maintenance of an ALI, the integration of multiple cell types, and the scalability of the culture system. Addressing these challenges is crucial for advancing the field of lung organoid research and maximizing the potential of these models for scientific discovery and therapeutic development.

The challenge of vascularization in lung organoids is a significant hurdle in the field of tissue engineering, as it is crucial for providing nutrients, oxygen, and removing waste to maintain tissue viability and function. Researchers have been developing innovative strategies to address this issue, aiming to create a more accurate representation of the lung's complex vasculature within organoids.

One approach involves the co-culture of lung organoids with endothelial cells, which are the cells that line blood vessels. By incorporating these cells into the organoid structure, scientists can encourage the formation of blood vessel-like structures, enhancing the organoid's resemblance to actual lung tissue. This method not only improves the delivery of nutrients and oxygen but also allows for the study of interactions between lung cells and blood vessels, which is critical for understanding various lung diseases and developing treatments.

Another strategy is the use of microfluidic devices, which can simulate the flow of blood through small channels. These devices can be integrated with lung organoids to create a dynamic environment where fluids can be circulated, mimicking the blood flow in actual lung tissue. This setup enables researchers to study the effects of blood flow on lung cells and the organoid's overall function.

Bioprinting technology has also been employed to create lung organoids with vascular structures. By printing cells in a specific pattern, researchers can design organoids that include pathways for blood vessel formation. This precision allows for the creation of more complex organoid models that can be used for drug testing and disease modeling.

Some groups have attempted to vascularize lung organoids by transplanting them into host animals, such as mice. The host's circulatory system can infiltrate the organoid, providing it with a natural source of blood vessels. While this method can be effective, it raises ethical considerations and is not suitable for all types of research.

Advancements in stem cell technology have also contributed to the vascularization of lung organoids. Scientists can now derive vascular progenitor cells from stem cells and incorporate them into organoids. These progenitor cells have the potential to develop into fully functional blood vessels within the organoid structure.

Researchers are also exploring the use of decellularized lung tissue as a scaffold for growing lung organoids. This tissue retains the original vascular architecture of the lung, and when repopulated with lung cells, it can provide a pre-existing network of blood vessels for the organoid.

The development of vascularized lung organoids is still in its early stages, and there are many challenges to overcome. However, the progress made so far is promising, and continued research in this area could lead to more physiologically relevant organoid models that can be used for a wide range of applications, from studying lung development and disease to testing new drugs and therapies. As the field advances, it is likely that new techniques and approaches will emerge, further enhancing the ability to create vascularized lung organoids that closely mimic the structure and function of human lungs.

The current methods for vascularizing lung organoids, while innovative and promising, come with a set of limitations that researchers are actively working to overcome. One of the main challenges is the complexity of the lung's vascular network, which is difficult to replicate in vitro. The organoids lack the intricate capillary networks that are essential for efficient gas exchange and nutrient delivery in living lungs.

Another limitation is the difficulty in achieving full maturation and functionality of the blood vessel-like structures within the organoids. Even when endothelial cells are incorporated, they often do not form the tight junctions and barrier functions that are characteristic of true blood vessels. This can lead to inadequate perfusion and the inability to mimic the selective permeability required for proper lung function.

The reliance on host animals for in vivo vascularization raises ethical concerns and may introduce variables that are not present in human biology, potentially skewing research results. Additionally, the use of animal models limits the translational potential of the findings to human treatments and therapies.

Microfluidic devices, while useful for simulating blood flow, cannot fully replicate the dynamic interactions between blood vessels and lung tissue that occur in the body. These interactions are crucial for understanding diseases and developing treatments. Moreover, the scalability of these devices for high-throughput applications remains a challenge.

Bioprinting techniques, although precise, are still in their infancy and often result in vascular structures that lack the robustness and durability of natural vessels. The bio printed vessels may also have limited life spans, which can be a significant drawback for long-term studies.

The co-culture of organoids with endothelial cells or the use of stem cell-derived vascular progenitors requires fine-tuning to ensure proper integration and function of the vascular components. Achieving the correct balance of growth factors and signaling molecules is a delicate process that can be hard to standardize.

Decellularized lung tissue provides a pre-existing vascular scaffold, but the process of decellularization and subsequent recellularization can affect the mechanical properties and biological functionality of the tissue. There is also a risk of immunogenicity when using decellularized tissue from non-autologous sources.

Overall, while the methods for vascularizing lung organoids represent significant advancements in the field, they are not without their challenges. Researchers must continue to refine these techniques to create more accurate and functional models of the human lung. The development of fully vascularized lung organoids would be a monumental step forward, offering deeper insights into lung physiology and pathology and accelerating the discovery of new treatments for lung diseases.

Emerging approaches to address the limitations in vascularization of lung organoids are focusing on enhancing the complexity and functionality of the organoid models. Recent advancements include the development of co-culture systems that integrate lung organoids with endothelial cells to promote the formation of capillary-like structures within the organoids. This method aims to create a more physiologically relevant model by mimicking the lung's vascular network.

Another innovative approach is the use of microfluidic platforms, which allow for the precise control of fluid flow and the establishment of a dynamic environment that simulates the blood flow in the lung's vasculature. These platforms can be integrated with lung organoids to study the effects of vascularization on organoid growth and function.

Bioprinting technology is also being explored to address vascularization challenges. With bioprinting, it is possible to design and create three-dimensional structures with embedded vascular channels. This technique has the potential to produce lung organoids with pre-formed vascular networks, which could significantly improve nutrient and oxygen delivery within the organoids.

The introduction of precision gene editing tools has opened new possibilities for creating lung organoids with specific characteristics. By editing the genes of stem cells used to generate organoids, researchers can induce the formation of vascular structures or introduce markers that help in studying the interaction between lung cells and blood vessels.

Researchers are also investigating the use of functional hydrogels as scaffolds for lung organoids. These hydrogels can be engineered to contain growth factors and other signaling molecules that encourage the formation of vascular structures and support the maturation of lung cells within the organoids.

The implementation of compartmentalization techniques is another emerging approach. By creating distinct compartments within the organoid culture, scientists can control organoid-organoid communication and prevent uncontrolled fusion, which is crucial for maintaining the structural integrity of the vascular network.

Additionally, there is a growing interest in developing differentiation protocols for region-specific organoids. This would allow for the generation of lung organoids that more closely resemble specific areas of the lung, such as the alveoli or airways, and could lead to better models for studying diseases that affect these regions.

Standardization of organoid cultures through microwell-based approaches is also being pursued. This method could lead to more consistent and reproducible organoid cultures, which is essential for high-throughput screening and other large-scale applications.

In summary, the field of lung organoid research is rapidly evolving, with new techniques and strategies being developed to overcome the limitations of current vascularization methods. These emerging approaches are enhancing the physiological relevance of lung organoids, making them more valuable tools for studying lung biology, disease, and therapy development. As these technologies mature, they hold the promise of revolutionizing our understanding of lung function and pathology, leading to breakthroughs in the treatment of lung diseases.

Improved vascularization in lung organoids has profound implications for drug testing, significantly enhancing the predictive accuracy of preclinical studies. With better vascularization, organoids can more closely mimic the human lung's physiological conditions, which is crucial for evaluating the pharmacokinetics and pharmacodynamics of potential therapeutic agents. Enhanced vascular structures within the organoids allow for more efficient delivery and distribution of drugs, enabling researchers to observe more accurate drug responses and interactions at the cellular level.

This advancement also facilitates the study of drug metabolism and clearance, as the presence of a vascular network can simulate the removal of metabolites and drugs, akin to the process in a living organism. Consequently, drugs can be screened for their efficacy and toxicity in a more body-like environment, potentially reducing the failure rate of drugs when they proceed to clinical trials. Moreover, the improved maturation and complexities of vascularized organoids can extend the culture time, allowing for long-term studies of drug effects and the development of resistance, which is particularly relevant for chronic treatments.

The implications extend to personalized medicine as well. Vascularized lung organoids can be derived from patient-specific cells, providing a platform for individualized drug response testing. This means that the efficacy and side effects of drugs can be tested on organoids that genetically match the patient, paving the way for more tailored and effective treatments. This approach could revolutionize the treatment of diseases like lung cancer, where the genetic makeup of the tumor significantly influences the response to various therapies.

Furthermore, the ability to test drugs on vascularized organoids may reduce the reliance on animal testing, aligning with the ethical push towards reducing animal use in research. It also addresses the translational gap between animal models and human patients, as drugs that are effective in animals do not always translate to human success due to physiological differences.

In the realm of infectious diseases, vascularized lung organoids could provide insights into how respiratory pathogens interact with the vasculature and how this interaction affects the efficacy of antiviral and antibiotic treatments. Understanding these dynamics is crucial for developing treatments for diseases like COVID-19, which affects both the respiratory tract and the vascular system.

The development of vascularized lung organoids also holds promise for the study of lung diseases that specifically affect the vasculature, such as pulmonary hypertension. By providing a model to study the disease in a controlled environment, researchers can gain insights into pathophysiology and explore potential therapeutic targets.

In summary, the implications of improved vascularization for drug testing using lung organoids are vast and transformative. This technological leap forward offers the potential for more accurate drug screening, personalized medicine, reduced animal testing, and a deeper understanding of lung physiology and pathology. As technology continues to evolve, it will likely become an indispensable tool in the development of new and more effective treatments for lung diseases.

Validating that drug responses in vascularized organoids correlate with human patient outcomes is a multifaceted process that involves several steps to ensure the organoids' clinical relevance. Initially, researchers must establish that the organoid models accurately recapitulate the structural and functional characteristics of the target human tissue. This is achieved through rigorous comparison of the organoids' genomic, transcriptomic, and proteomic profiles with those of the original patient samples.

Once the organoids are confirmed to be representative of the human condition, researchers can proceed with drug testing. This involves exposing the organoids to various pharmacological agents and observing the responses, such as changes in cell viability, morphology, and gene expression. These responses are then compared to clinical data from patients who have received the same treatments, looking for correlations in efficacy and adverse effects.

Another critical aspect of validation is the use of high-throughput screening techniques to test a wide range of drugs and dosages on the organoids. This allows for the collection of extensive data that can be analyzed using bioinformatics tools to identify patterns and predict patient outcomes. The results from these screenings can be cross-referenced with patient databases to find matches and validate the organoids' predictive power.

Longitudinal studies are also essential, where organoids derived from patients at different stages of treatment are monitored over time. This approach helps in understanding the evolution of drug responses and resistance mechanisms, which can be compared with the patients' clinical progression to validate the organoids' utility in predicting long-term outcomes.

In addition to these methods, researchers are exploring the integration of vascularized organoids with microfluidic systems that simulate the human circulatory system. This innovation allows for a more dynamic and systemic evaluation of drug responses, including the study of pharmacokinetics and pharmacodynamics, which are crucial for predicting how drugs will behave in the human body.

Furthermore, the development of standardized protocols for organoid generation and drug testing is vital for validation. Standardization ensures that the results are reproducible and comparable across different studies, which is necessary for establishing the organoids as reliable models for predicting patient outcomes.

Collaboration with clinical trials is another avenue for validation. By comparing organoid-based predictions with outcomes from clinical trials, researchers can directly assess the accuracy of the organoids in a real-world setting. This also provides an opportunity to refine the organoid models based on clinical feedback.

Lastly, the incorporation of machine learning algorithms can enhance the validation process. These algorithms can analyze complex datasets from organoid screenings and clinical trials to identify correlations and make predictions about patient outcomes. The use of artificial intelligence in this context can significantly improve the precision and reliability of organoid-based drug testing.

In conclusion, the validation of drug responses in vascularized organoids as correlates for human patient outcomes is a comprehensive process that requires a combination of advanced technologies, standardized methodologies, and collaborative efforts between researchers and clinicians. As the field progresses, these validation strategies will continue to evolve, further cementing the role of organoids in personalized medicine and drug development.

The field of personalized medicine has been significantly advanced using patient-derived organoids (PDOs), which have shown promising results in correlating organoid responses with patient outcomes. For instance, a study highlighted in a consensus on organoid-based drug sensitivity testing for cancer precision medicine demonstrated a strong correlation between clinical outcomes and the efficacy of chemotherapy and/or radiotherapy predicted by PDOs. This suggests that organoids can be reliable predictors of how a patient might respond to certain cancer treatments.

In another example, the TUMOROID study utilized organoids derived from metastatic colorectal cancer (CRC) patients and found that the organoid treatment response was able to predict the response to irinotecan-based therapies in more than 80% of patients without misclassifying those who responded to the treatment. This level of accuracy is particularly noteworthy as it indicates that organoids can be a powerful tool in determining the most effective treatment for patients, potentially leading to better outcomes and personalized therapy plans.

Moreover, molecular profiling of tumor organoids has been matched with drug-screening results, suggesting that patient-derived organoids could complement existing approaches in defining cancer vulnerabilities and improving treatment responses. This approach allows for a more targeted and efficient way to identify potential treatments that are more likely to be successful in individual patients, thereby reducing the time and cost associated with traditional trial-and-error methods.

These examples underscore the potential of organoids as a transformative technology in the realm of drug testing and treatment response prediction. As the technology continues to develop and more studies are conducted, it is likely that the use of organoids will become more widespread in clinical settings, offering hope for more effective and personalized treatments for patients across a variety of diseases. The success of these correlations not only validates the use of organoids in research but also paves the way for their integration into routine clinical practice, marking a significant step forward in the journey towards truly personalized medicine. The implications of these findings are vast, with the potential to revolutionize how we approach the treatment of cancer and other complex diseases.

Implementing organoid-based predictions in clinical practice is a complex endeavor that faces several challenges. One of the primary issues is the need for rapid and efficient generation of patient-derived organoids (PDOs) from limited tumor material, which is often the case in clinical settings. This requires not only technical expertise but also the development of standardized protocols that can be applied across different laboratories and institutions.

Another significant challenge is the testing of a broad panel of anti-cancer drugs on PDOs. This is essential for identifying the most effective treatment for a patient, but it demands extensive resources and can be time-consuming. Moreover, the results must be obtained within a timeframe that is compatible with the urgent needs of patient disease management. Delays in obtaining results could render the organoid-based predictions irrelevant if the patient's condition progresses too rapidly.

The variability in organoid formation and drug response is another hurdle. High variations can reduce the reproducibility and reliability of the results, which is critical when making clinical decisions based on these predictions. Researchers must find ways to minimize this variability to ensure that the organoid-based predictions are consistent and can be trusted by clinicians.

Furthermore, the organoid technology must comprehensively reflect intra-tumor heterogeneity and the tumor microenvironment, including tumor angiogenesis. These factors are crucial for accurately predicting how a tumor will respond to treatment, yet they are challenging to replicate in vitro. Developing organoids that can capture this complexity is an ongoing area of research.

Reducing research costs is also a concern, as the development and maintenance of organoid cultures can be expensive. This can limit the accessibility of organoid-based predictions in clinical practice, particularly in resource-limited settings. Finding cost-effective methods to generate and use organoids is essential for broader implementation.

Lastly, there is a need for standardized construction processes while retaining reliability. Standardization can facilitate the comparison of results across different studies and institutions, but it must not come at the expense of the organoids' ability to accurately model individual patient tumors. Balancing standardization with customization is a delicate task that researchers and clinicians must navigate as they work towards integrating organoid-based predictions into routine clinical practice.

In summary, while organoid-based predictions hold great promise for personalized medicine, the challenges in implementing them in clinical practice are significant. They encompass technical, logistical, and economic aspects, all of which must be addressed to realize the full potential of this innovative approach to cancer treatment and drug development. As the field advances, collaboration between researchers, clinicians, and policymakers will be crucial in overcoming these obstacles and bringing the benefits of organoid technology to patients.

The integration of organoid-based predictions into existing clinical workflows is a multifaceted process that requires careful planning and coordination across various levels of healthcare delivery. A consensus-driven approach is essential for the successful adoption of this technology, ensuring that all stakeholders, including clinicians, researchers, and laboratory technicians, are aligned in their understanding and application of organoid-based drug sensitivity testing (DST).

To begin with, clear guidelines and protocols need to be established for the generation, characterization, and use of patient-derived organoids (PDOs). These guidelines should cover the entire process, from tissue sampling and organoid culture to drug testing and data interpretation. Standardization of these protocols is crucial for ensuring reproducibility and reliability of results across different settings.

Once the protocols are in place, training programs should be developed to equip healthcare professionals with the necessary skills to implement organoid-based DST. This includes understanding the principles behind organoid culture, the nuances of drug testing on these models, and the interpretation of results in the context of patient care.

The next step involves the integration of organoid-based DST into the laboratory diagnostic tests (LDTs) that are routinely used in clinical practice. This requires the establishment of laboratory infrastructure capable of supporting organoid culture and testing, as well as the development of data management systems to handle the complex information generated by these tests.

Clinical decision support systems (CDSS) can play a pivotal role in integrating organoid-based predictions into clinical workflows. These systems can analyze organoid testing results alongside patient data to provide clinicians with evidence-based treatment recommendations. The CDSS should be designed to interface seamlessly with electronic health records (EHRs), allowing for a smooth integration of organoid-based data into the patient's overall care plan.

Collaboration with regulatory bodies is also essential to ensure that organoid-based DST meets the necessary standards for clinical use. This includes obtaining the appropriate certifications and approvals for the use of organoids as a diagnostic tool, as well as establishing quality control measures to maintain the integrity of the testing process.

Furthermore, clinical trials are necessary to validate the efficacy and utility of organoid-based predictions in a real-world setting. These trials can provide the evidence needed to support the clinical adoption of organoid technology and demonstrate its impact on patient outcomes.

Patient engagement is another critical aspect of integrating organoid-based predictions into clinical practice. Patients should be informed about the benefits and limitations of organoid-based DST, and their consent should be obtained before using their tissue samples for organoid generation. Clear communication about the potential impact of organoid testing on treatment decisions is vital for patient acceptance and trust.

Finally, ongoing research and development are needed to continuously improve organoid technology and its application in clinical settings. This includes exploring new methods for organoid vascularization, enhancing the representation of tumor heterogeneity, and developing more sophisticated models for drug testing.

In summary, the integration of organoid-based predictions into clinical workflows is a complex but achievable goal. It requires a coordinated effort involving standardization, training, infrastructure development, regulatory collaboration, clinical validation, patient engagement, and continuous research. With these elements in place, organoid-based DST has the potential to significantly improve personalized medicine and enhance the quality of care for patients with various diseases.

Unlocking Next-Gen Antibiotics:

An international research effort has identified almost a million potential sources of antibiotics in the natural world. This discovery could pave the way for novel antibiotic development.

The quest for next-generation antibiotics has taken a significant leap forward thanks to an international research team's groundbreaking discovery. By harnessing the power of machine learning, the team has identified an astonishing 863,498 potential sources of antibiotics from the natural world. This extensive study, published in the prestigious journal Cell, was spearheaded by Associate Professor Luis Pedro Coelho of Queensland University of Technology (QUT), as part of his ARC Future Fellowship. The research, which is a collaborative effort involving the University of Pennsylvania, Fudan University, the European Molecular Biology Laboratory, and APC Microbiome Ireland, represents a crucial step in combating the looming threat of antimicrobial resistance (AMR).

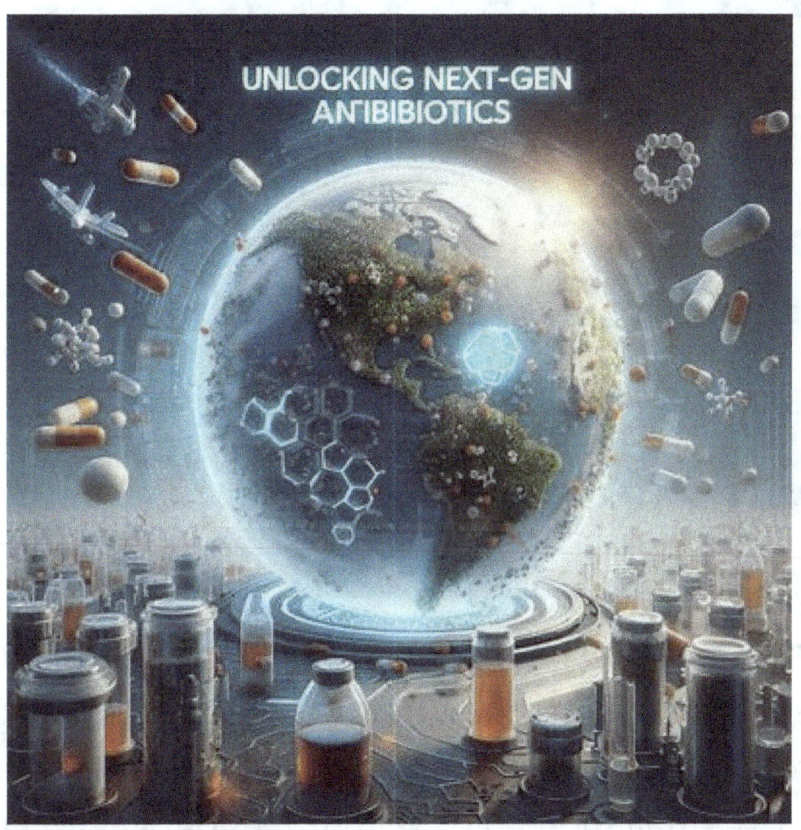

AMR poses one of the top public health threats globally, with an estimated 1.27 million deaths annually attributed to it. Without innovative interventions, AMR could result in up to 10 million deaths per year by 2050. The study's findings are timely, as the world grapples with an increasing number of superbugs that are resistant to existing drugs. The research team's approach involved analyzing over 60,000 metagenomes, which collectively contain the genetic material of more than one million organisms. These metagenomes were sourced from diverse environments across the globe, including marine and soil ecosystems, as well as human and animal guts.

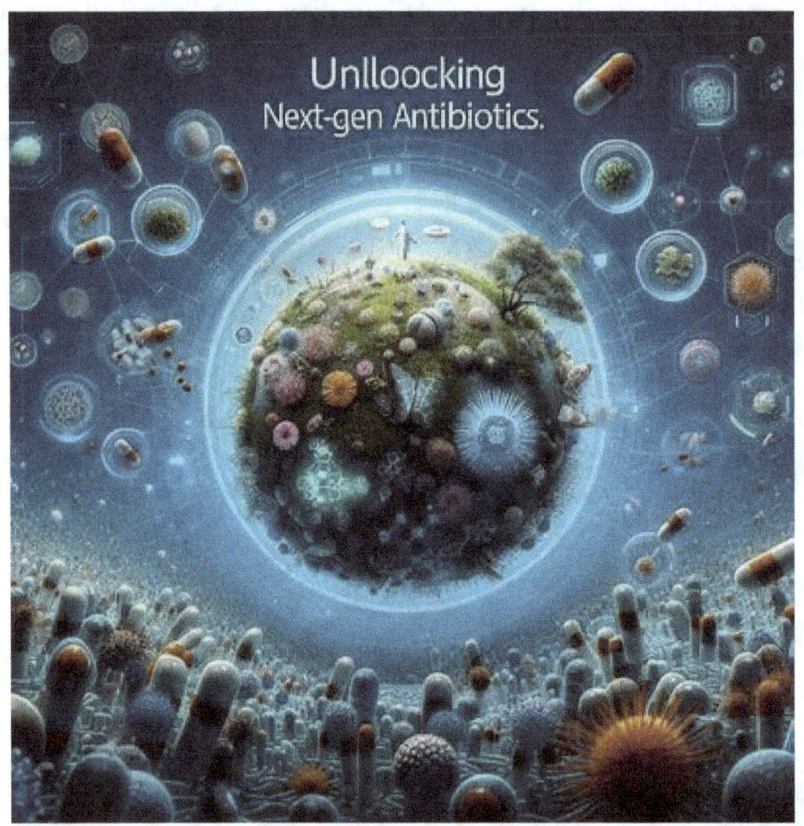

The team's use of artificial intelligence to sift through this vast amount of data is particularly noteworthy. Machine learning algorithms were employed to identify promising antimicrobial peptides (AMPs)—small molecules with the capability to kill or inhibit the growth of infectious microbes. The potential of these AMPs was then verified through laboratory tests, where 100 synthesized peptides were pitted against clinically significant pathogens. The results were promising: 79 of these peptides disrupted bacterial membranes, and 63 targeted antibiotic-resistant bacteria such as Staphylococcus aureus and Escherichia coli.

Some of the peptides even demonstrated the ability to eliminate infections in mice models, with two peptides reducing bacterial presence by up to four orders of magnitude. These results are comparable to the effects of polymyxin B, a commercially available antibiotic used to treat serious infections like meningitis, pneumonia, sepsis, and urinary tract infections.

The culmination of this research is the creation of AMPSphere—a comprehensive database comprising these novel peptides. AMPSphere stands as a publicly available, open-access resource, poised to catalyze further antibiotic discovery and development. By making this database accessible to researchers worldwide, the team has provided a valuable tool that could lead to the creation of new antibiotics, offering hope in the fight against the ever-growing challenge of antibiotic-resistant bacteria.

Antimicrobial peptides (AMPs), also known as host defense peptides, are small, naturally occurring molecules that play a crucial role in the innate immune system of various organisms. These peptides are typically composed of 10 to 60 amino acids and are characterized by their broad-spectrum activity against a wide range of pathogens, including bacteria, viruses, fungi, and even cancer cells. AMPs are unique in their mode of action; they can directly kill microbes by disrupting their cell membranes or by interfering with their internal machinery. Unlike traditional antibiotics, which often target specific bacterial functions and can lead to resistance, AMPs offer a more general attack, making it harder for microbes to develop resistance.

The structure of AMPs is key to their function. They are amphipathic, meaning they have both hydrophilic (water-attracting) and hydrophobic (water-repelling) properties. This allows them to integrate into microbial membranes, which are also amphipathic, and disrupt their integrity. Some AMPs can form pores in the membranes, leading to cell death, while others might penetrate the cell to interact with intracellular targets. Additionally, AMPs can also modulate the host's immune response, enhancing the body's ability to fight off infections.

The potential of AMPs extends beyond their antimicrobial properties. Research has shown that they can have immunomodulatory effects, which means they can influence the immune system to enhance its response to infections. This dual action makes AMPs particularly valuable as therapeutic agents. In the context of increasing antibiotic resistance, AMPs are being studied as a promising alternative to traditional antibiotics. They could be used not only to treat infections but also to prevent them, especially in clinical settings where the risk of infection is high.

The discovery and development of new AMPs are ongoing areas of research. Scientists are exploring various natural sources, including plants, animals, and even human tissues, to find new peptides with potent antimicrobial properties. Advances in biotechnology have also allowed for the synthetic creation of

AMPs, which can be designed to have specific characteristics, such as increased stability or targeted activity against pathogens.

In summary, antimicrobial peptides are a vital part of our defense against microbial infections. Their broad-spectrum activity, combined with their ability to evade resistance, makes them an exciting area of research and a potential cornerstone of future antimicrobial therapies.

Antimicrobial peptides (AMPs) and traditional antibiotics represent two distinct classes of antimicrobial agents, each with unique features and mechanisms of action. AMPs are small molecules that are part of the innate immune system of all living organisms, providing a first line of defense against pathogens. They are known for their broad-spectrum activity, which allows them to target a wide range of microorganisms, including bacteria, viruses, fungi, and even some cancer cells. One of the key differences between AMPs and traditional antibiotics is their mode of action. AMPs typically work by disrupting the cell membranes of pathogens, leading to rapid cell death. This mechanism is less specific than that of traditional antibiotics, which often target particular bacterial processes or structures, such as protein synthesis or cell wall formation.

Another significant difference is the rate at which resistance develops. Traditional antibiotics, due to their specific targets, can lead to the development of resistance as bacteria evolve mechanisms to circumvent the drug's action. In contrast, because

AMPs disrupt cell membranes, a fundamental component of microbial cells, it is more challenging for pathogens to develop resistance against them. Additionally, AMPs can also modulate the immune response, enhancing the body's natural ability to fight infections, which is not a feature of most traditional antibiotics.

The structure of AMPs is also distinct; they are typically amphipathic, meaning they possess both hydrophilic and hydrophobic properties, allowing them to integrate into and disrupt microbial membranes. Traditional antibiotics do not share this amphipathic nature. Furthermore, AMPs are generally smaller and have a wider variety of structures compared to traditional antibiotics, which tend to have more uniform and larger molecular structures.

The development of AMPs as therapeutic agents is driven by the urgent need to combat antibiotic-resistant bacteria. While traditional antibiotics have saved countless lives since their discovery, their overuse and misuse have led to the rise of resistant strains of bacteria, making some infections difficult to treat. AMPs offer a promising alternative due to their potent antimicrobial properties and lower likelihood of resistance development.

In summary, AMPs differ from traditional antibiotics in their broad-spectrum activity, mode of action, structure, and the way they interact with the immune system. These differences make AMPs a valuable addition to the arsenal of antimicrobial agents, especially in the face of increasing antibiotic resistance.

Antimicrobial peptides (AMPs) have emerged as a promising complement to traditional antibiotics, offering a potential solution to the growing challenge of antibiotic resistance. The unique mechanisms of action of AMPs, which include disrupting cell membranes and modulating immune responses, make them suitable candidates for combination therapy with conventional antibiotics. This synergistic approach can enhance the effectiveness of treatment and reduce the likelihood of resistance development.

The use of AMPs alongside traditional antibiotics is based on the concept of combination therapy, which involves using two or more drugs with different mechanisms of action to treat an infection. This strategy can be particularly effective against multi-drug resistant pathogens, as it can limit the ability of bacteria to adapt and survive. Studies have shown that when AMPs are used in conjunction with antibiotics, they can help to break down bacterial defenses, making the bacteria more susceptible to the antibiotics' effects.

Moreover, AMPs can target a broader range of bacterial functions compared to traditional antibiotics, which often focus on a single target, such as protein synthesis or cell wall formation. By attacking multiple sites within the bacteria, AMPs can weaken the bacteria's overall structure and function, allowing antibiotics to work more effectively. Additionally, AMPs can disrupt biofilms, which are protective layers that bacteria form to shield themselves from antibiotics. When used together, AMPs can penetrate these biofilms, enabling antibiotics to reach and eliminate the bacteria hidden within.

The potential of AMPs to enhance antibiotic therapy has been recognized in clinical settings, where researchers are exploring their use as adjuvants to existing treatments. For instance, some AMPs have been found to restore the efficacy of antibiotics that bacteria had previously become resistant to. This is particularly important in hospital environments, where antibiotic-resistant infections are a significant concern.

Furthermore, the combination of AMPs and antibiotics can lead to a reduction in the dosage of antibiotics required, potentially minimizing side effects and the risk of toxicity. This is beneficial for patients, especially those who are vulnerable or have compromised immune systems. It also contributes to the global effort to reduce the overuse of antibiotics, which is a key factor in the development of resistance.

In conclusion, the integration of AMPs with traditional antibiotics represents a promising avenue in the fight against antibiotic-resistant infections. By combining the broad-spectrum activity of AMPs with the targeted action of antibiotics, healthcare providers can offer more effective and potentially safer treatments. As research progresses, it is likely that we will see an increase in the clinical application of AMPs in combination with antibiotics, providing a new weapon in the battle against the superbugs of the future.

Antimicrobial peptides (AMPs) are increasingly being recognized for their potential in combination therapy with traditional antibiotics to enhance antimicrobial efficacy and reduce resistance. One notable example is the use of colistin, a polypeptide antibiotic that disrupts bacterial cell membranes, in combination with rifampicin, which inhibits RNA synthesis. This combination has been effective against multi-drug resistant strains of Pseudomonas aeruginosa and Acinetobacter baumannii. Another example is the combination of daptomycin, an AMP that disrupts cell membrane integrity, with β-lactam antibiotics like ceftobiprole, which inhibit cell wall synthesis. This combination has shown synergistic effects against methicillin-resistant Staphylococcus aureus (MRSA).

Furthermore, research has demonstrated the effectiveness of combining AMP pexiganan, which has a broad spectrum of activity, with the antibiotic tobramycin to treat Pseudomonas aeruginosa infections. Pexiganan disrupts the bacterial cell membrane, while tobramycin inhibits protein synthesis. Similarly, the AMP LL-37, which is derived from human cathelicidin and has immunomodulatory properties, has been used in conjunction with vancomycin, enhancing its activity against vancomycin-resistant enterococci.

In addition to these, the peptide nisin, produced by Lactococcus lactis, has been used alongside antibiotics like penicillin and chloramphenicol to combat Streptococcus pneumoniae. Nisin forms pores in bacterial cell membranes, which can increase the susceptibility of bacteria to other antibiotics. Another AMP, polymyxin B, has been used with meropenem, a carbapenem antibiotic, to treat infections caused by carbapenem-resistant Enterobacteriaceae.

The combination of AMPs with traditional antibiotics is not limited to treating bacterial infections; some AMPs have also been used alongside antifungal agents. For instance, the AMP histatin-5, which targets fungal cell walls, has been combined with fluconazole, an inhibitor of fungal cell membrane synthesis, to treat Candida infections.

These examples illustrate the versatility and potential of AMPs in combination therapy. By targeting different aspects of microbial physiology, AMPs can work synergistically with antibiotics to enhance their efficacy, reduce the required dosage, and minimize the development of resistance. As research continues, it is expected that more AMPs will be identified and utilized in combination therapies to address the growing challenge of antimicrobial resistance.

Determining the optimal combination of antimicrobial peptides (AMPs) and antibiotics is a complex process that involves a multifaceted approach, combining experimental research with advanced computational methods. Researchers start by identifying potential AMPs and antibiotics that could work well together, based on their known mechanisms of action and spectrum of activity. They then conduct in vitro tests, such as checkerboard assays, to assess the interactions between different combinations of AMPs and antibiotics. These assays help determine whether the combinations are synergistic, additive, or antagonistic in their effects against specific pathogens.

Synergy is particularly sought after, as it implies that the combination is more effective than the sum of its parts. To quantify this, researchers measure the minimum inhibitory concentrations (MICs) of each agent alone and in combination. A decrease in the MICs when used together indicates a synergistic interaction. Furthermore, time-kill assays are performed to observe the rate at which bacteria are killed by the combination, providing insights into the efficacy and potential clinical application of the combination.

Advanced computational methods, such as machine learning algorithms, are increasingly being utilized to predict the synergistic effects of AMPs and antibiotics. These algorithms can process large datasets, including the properties of AMPs and antibiotics, their MICs, and the characteristics of target pathogens, to predict which combinations are likely to be effective. This approach can significantly reduce the time and resources required for experimental studies by narrowing down the most promising combinations for further testing.

Researchers also consider the pharmacodynamics and pharmacokinetics of the drugs, which involve the drugs' interactions with the body and the pathogens, respectively. This includes studying the absorption, distribution, metabolism, and excretion of the drugs, as well as their post-antibiotic effects. Animal models are often used to study these aspects in a living organism, providing a more accurate prediction of how the combination will perform in humans.

Another critical factor is the potential for toxicity and side effects. Researchers must ensure that the combination of AMPs and antibiotics does not produce harmful effects that outweigh the benefits of the treatment. This involves conducting cytotoxicity assays and evaluating the safety profile of the drug combination in cell cultures and animal models before proceeding to clinical trials.

Finally, the clinical context in which the combination will be used is considered. This includes the site of infection, the patient population, and the presence of any underlying conditions that may affect the treatment's efficacy or safety. Researchers aim to develop combinations that are not only effective against pathogens but also suitable for use in diverse clinical scenarios.

In summary, the determination of the optimal combination of AMPs and antibiotics is a rigorous process that integrates experimental data with computational predictions, pharmacological studies, and clinical considerations. This comprehensive approach ensures that the combinations developed are both effective against pathogens and safe for patients, ultimately contributing to the advancement of antimicrobial therapy.

The exploration of antimicrobial peptides (AMPs) in combination with traditional antibiotics is a burgeoning field, with several clinical trials underway to evaluate the efficacy and safety of such treatments. One of the most promising studies is being conducted by the Ineos Oxford Institute (IOI), where scientists have discovered a novel triple drug combination that targets two key bacterial enzymes involved in resistance. This combination includes the β-lactam antibiotic meropenem, a newly developed metallo-β-lactamase (MBL) inhibitor called indole-2-carboxylate 58 (InC58), and a serine-β-lactamase (SBL) inhibitor known as avibactam (AVI). The study, which has been published in the journal Engineering, aims to combat antimicrobial resistance (AMR) by simultaneously addressing multiple resistance mechanisms.

Another significant trial is a systematic review of clinical studies focusing on the treatment of severe infections caused by carbapenem-resistant gram-negative bacteria. This review aims to critically evaluate all available antibiotic options for such infections, with a particular focus on combination therapies. Additionally, recent studies have highlighted the effectiveness of cationic AMPs, such as LL-37, in combination with various antibiotics like polymyxin E and piperacillin, against highly multidrug-resistant gram-negative and methicillin-resistant Staphylococcus aureus (MRSA) pathogens.

Furthermore, the clinical pipeline as of December 2022 includes several β-lactamase inhibitor (BLI) combinations that are being evaluated in phase I, II, or III clinical trials. These trials are investigating the development status, mode of action, spectra of activity, and origins of these compounds, whether they are natural products, synthetic, or protein/mammalian peptides. A novel approach consisting of collaborative filtering, link prediction, and AMP feature analysis has also been developed to predict previously unknown, bacteria-specific activity of AMP combinations, suggest novel synergistic AMP-antibiotic combinations, and guide the future design of effective AMP-AMP combinations.

These clinical trials and studies represent a concerted effort by the scientific community to address the pressing issue of AMR. By exploring the synergistic potential of AMPs and antibiotics, researchers hope to develop new therapeutic strategies that can overcome the limitations of current treatments and provide more effective solutions for patients suffering from resistant infections. The outcomes of these trials could have a profound impact on the future of antimicrobial therapy, offering new hope in the battle against some of the most challenging bacterial adversaries. As these trials progress, they will provide valuable data that can inform clinical practices and potentially lead to the introduction of new combination therapies into standard medical care. The ongoing research and development in this area underscore the importance of innovation and collaboration in the fight against AMR, ensuring that healthcare providers continue to have effective tools at their disposal to treat infections in an ever-evolving landscape of microbial resistance.

In clinical trials evaluating antimicrobial peptide (AMP)-antibiotic combinations, the specific endpoints are critical for determining the efficacy and safety of the treatment. These endpoints typically include measures of clinical effectiveness, such as all-cause mortality, attributable mortality, and improvement in clinical parameters or specific biomarkers. Microbiological eradication, which assesses the complete elimination of the targeted pathogen, is another common endpoint. Researchers also look at antibiotic- or organ-failure-free days to evaluate the broader health impacts of the treatment. Quality of life evaluations are included to assess the treatment's effect on patients' well-being.

Furthermore, the trials may monitor for the development of resistance, both in the short term and over a more extended period, to ensure that the combination therapy does not contribute to the growing problem of antimicrobial resistance (AMR). Safety endpoints, such as the incidence of adverse reactions and toxicity levels, are also crucial to ensure that the combination therapy is not only effective but also safe for patients. In some cases, surrogate endpoints may be used to predict clinical outcomes based on physiological or laboratory measurements.

The choice of endpoints often depends on the phase of the trial. Early-phase trials might focus more on safety and pharmacokinetics, while later-phase trials prioritize clinical outcomes and long-term effects. The endpoints are selected to provide the most comprehensive understanding of the treatment's impact, ensuring that the benefits outweigh any potential risks.

In addition to these standard endpoints, some trials may include innovative measures such as the use of advanced imaging techniques or genetic markers to provide deeper insights into the treatment's mechanisms of action and effects. These can help to identify which patients are most likely to benefit from the therapy and to tailor treatments to individual needs.

Overall, the endpoints in these clinical trials are designed to rigorously evaluate the potential of AMP-antibiotic combinations to provide a new solution in the fight against resistant infections. By carefully selecting and measuring these endpoints, researchers can ensure that the results of the trials are robust, reliable, and relevant to clinical practice.

Microbiological eradication in clinical trials is defined as the complete elimination of the targeted pathogen from the body, as evidenced by repeated negative cultures from the site of infection. This outcome is crucial for determining the efficacy of antimicrobial treatments, including those involving antimicrobial peptides (AMPs) and traditional antibiotics. To establish microbiological eradication, researchers collect samples from the infected area before and after treatment. A post-treatment culture that shows no growth of the initial pathogen indicates that microbiological eradication has been achieved. However, in some cases where it's not possible to obtain post-baseline culture results, such as in complicated intra-abdominal infections, presumed microbiological eradication may be assessed based on the resolution of clinical signs and symptoms.

Additionally, the definition encompasses not only the absence of the original pathogen but also considers the potential for relapse or superinfection. Relapse is defined as the re-isolation of the initial pathogen from the original site of infection after it was previously eradicated, with or without clinical deterioration. Superinfection refers to the isolation of a new pathogen that does not present at baseline. These factors are important for understanding the long-term effectiveness of the treatment and the patient's overall recovery.

In respiratory tract infections, for example, the need for bacterial eradication has been a subject of debate. However, evidence supports that active bacterial eradication is an important aim of antimicrobial therapy, as failure to eradicate bacteria may promote the emergence and dissemination of antimicrobial-resistant clones. In urinary tract infections, microbiological success might be defined as a reduction in the density of the original pathogen to a specific threshold on urine culture.

The primary outcome measures in trials often include clinical cure at the end of treatment and the test of cure (TOC) within the intention-to-treat (ITT) population, alongside the eradication of microbial infection at the end of antibiotic treatment in the ITT population. These endpoints help to ensure that the treatment not only addresses the symptoms but also effectively clears the infection, reducing the risk of recurrence and the spread of resistance.

Overall, the definition of microbiological eradication is a key component in the design and evaluation of clinical trials for antimicrobial therapies. It provides a clear and measurable outcome that reflects the direct impact of the treatment on the pathogen, contributing to the body of evidence needed to support the use of new and existing antimicrobial agents in clinical practice.

In microbiological eradication studies, researchers account for the presence of biofilms by employing a variety of strategies that address the unique challenges posed by these complex microbial communities. Biofilms are structured aggregates of microorganisms that are embedded within a self-produced matrix of extracellular polymeric substances (EPS), which confer protection against antimicrobial agents and the host immune system. To effectively study biofilm-associated infections and their eradication, researchers must consider the biofilm's resilience and its distinct physiological state compared to planktonic (free-floating) bacteria.

One approach is the use of in vitro biofilm models that mimic the natural environment of biofilms, allowing for the study of biofilm formation, structure, and response to antimicrobial treatments. These models can range from simple static cultures to more sophisticated flow cell systems that simulate the fluid dynamics of the human body. By using these models, scientists can observe the penetration of antibiotics into the biofilm and evaluate the efficacy of different antimicrobial agents.

Another important aspect is the selection of relevant endpoints that specifically measure biofilm eradication. Traditional microbiological assays, such as colony-forming unit (CFU) counts, may not be sufficient, as biofilm cells can be viable but non-culturable. Therefore, researchers often employ advanced techniques like confocal laser scanning microscopy (CLSM) combined with viability stains to visualize and quantify live and dead cells within the biofilm structure.

Researchers also focus on the development and testing of biofilm-specific antimicrobial agents, including those that can disrupt the EPS matrix, enhance the penetration of antibiotics, or target biofilm-specific metabolic pathways. Enzymes that degrade the EPS, quorum sensing inhibitors that prevent cell-to-cell communication, and bacteriophages that can penetrate and disrupt biofilms are examples of such agents.

Moreover, the study of biofilm eradication often involves the assessment of biofilm dispersal agents, which can detach biofilm cells and make them more susceptible to antibiotics. The effectiveness of these agents is evaluated in combination with antibiotics to determine if they can enhance treatment outcomes.

In clinical settings, researchers must also consider the impact of the host's immune system on biofilm eradication. The immune response can be both beneficial, by aiding in the removal of biofilm cells, and detrimental, by causing tissue damage. Therefore, studies often include the evaluation of the host-pathogen interaction and the role of the immune system in biofilm clearance.

Finally, researchers are exploring innovative treatment strategies, such as the use of antimicrobial peptides (AMPs), which have shown promise in targeting biofilm-associated infections. AMPs can disrupt microbial membranes and have been found to be effective against biofilm-forming bacteria. The potential of AMPs in combination with traditional antibiotics is a particularly exciting area of research, offering new possibilities for overcoming the challenges posed by biofilms.

In summary, accounting for the presence of biofilms in microbiological eradication studies involves a comprehensive approach that includes the use of appropriate in vitro models, the selection of biofilm-specific endpoints, the development of targeted antimicrobial agents, the assessment of biofilm dispersal strategies, the consideration of host immune responses, and the exploration of novel treatment options like AMPs. These efforts are crucial for advancing our understanding of biofilm-associated infections and developing effective strategies for their eradication. The ongoing research in this field is essential for addressing the significant clinical challenge posed by biofilms and improving outcomes for patients with biofilm-mediated infections.

Translating biofilm research findings into clinical practice involves navigating a complex landscape of challenges that span scientific, regulatory, and practical domains. One of the primary hurdles is the inherent complexity of biofilms themselves; these structured communities of microorganisms exhibit behaviors and resistance mechanisms that are significantly different from those of planktonic bacteria, making them difficult to study and target. In the laboratory, biofilms can be studied under controlled conditions, but these often fail to replicate the multifaceted environments found in clinical settings, where biofilms may interact with human tissues, medical devices, and a host of other factors.

Another significant challenge is the gap between the pace of scientific discovery and the slower process of clinical implementation. Research findings must undergo rigorous validation and testing before they can be applied in a healthcare setting, a process that can take years or even decades. This delay is exacerbated by the need for extensive clinical trials to ensure the safety and efficacy of new treatments derived from biofilm research.

Regulatory hurdles also play a role, as the approval process for new medical treatments is stringent and often requires a clear demonstration of benefit over existing therapies. Biofilm-related treatments must navigate these regulatory pathways, which can be both time-consuming and costly.

Moreover, there is a need for interdisciplinary collaboration to effectively translate biofilm research into practice. Researchers, clinicians, and industry professionals must work together to ensure that scientific insights are practically applicable and meet the needs of patients. However, differing priorities and communication barriers between these groups can impede progress.

The economic aspect cannot be overlooked either; developing new treatments from biofilm research requires significant investment, and there may be a lack of financial incentives for companies to pursue treatments that do not promise substantial profits. This is particularly true for antibiotic development, where the return on investment is often lower compared to other types of drugs.

Educational barriers also exist, as healthcare providers need to be informed about the latest research and how it can be integrated into their practice. Without adequate knowledge dissemination and training, even the most promising biofilm research findings may not be adopted by the medical community.

Lastly, the issue of antimicrobial resistance (AMR) adds another layer of complexity. As biofilms are known to contribute to AMR, any new treatments must be designed to not only be effective against biofilms but also to avoid contributing to the growing problem of resistant pathogens.

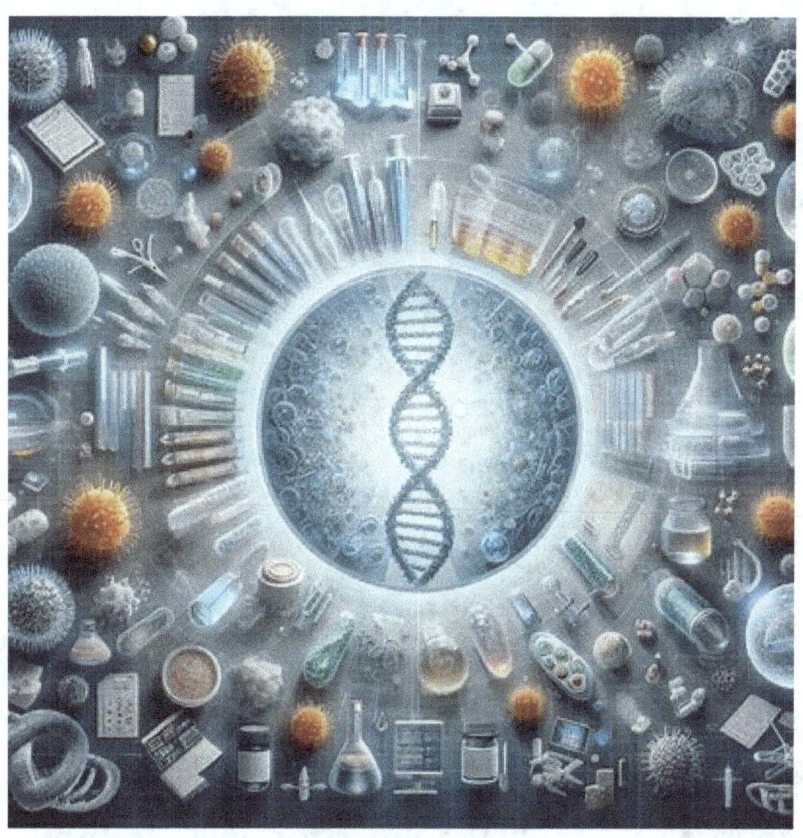

In summary, the translation of biofilm research into clinical practice is a multifaceted challenge that requires a concerted effort from researchers, clinicians, regulatory bodies, and industry stakeholders. Overcoming these obstacles is essential for harnessing the full potential of biofilm research to improve patient outcomes and combat the pressing issue of AMR. The development of frameworks and guidelines to facilitate this translation, as well as continued innovation and collaboration, will be key to bridging the gap between the laboratory and the clinic.

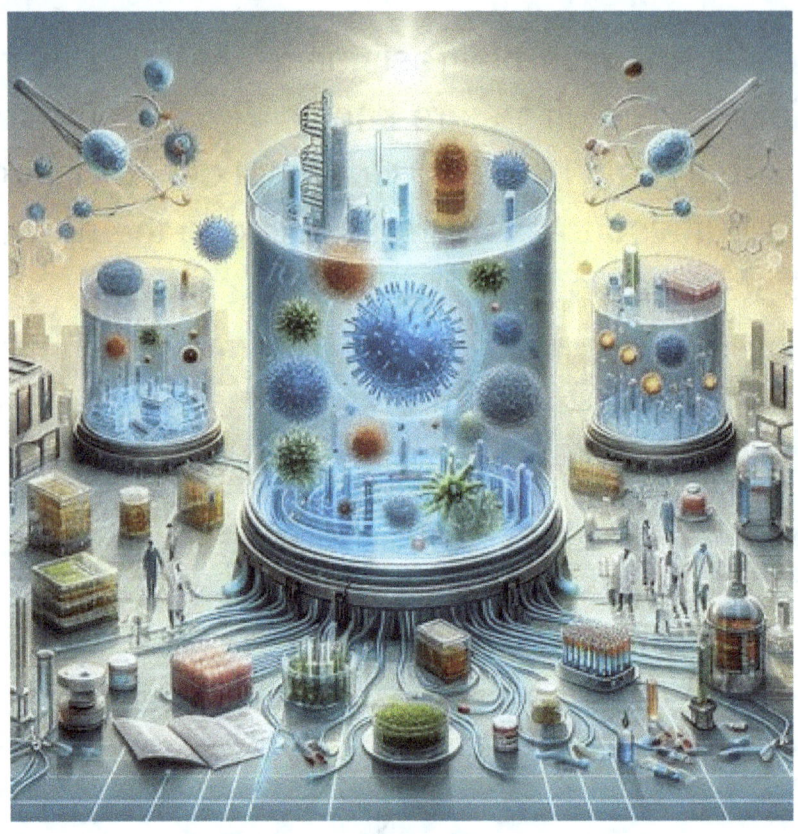

Healthcare institutions can employ a multifaceted approach to promote the adoption of biofilm-related treatments, which are crucial for enhancing patient outcomes and combating the persistent challenge of biofilm-associated infections. One effective strategy is to foster interdisciplinary collaboration among clinicians, researchers, and policymakers to facilitate the translation of research findings into clinical protocols. This can be achieved through the establishment of dedicated biofilm research and treatment centers that serve as hubs for innovation and education.

Education and training programs are also vital, as they can raise awareness about the significance of biofilms in clinical settings and disseminate knowledge on the latest biofilm management strategies. These programs should target not only healthcare providers but also patients, who can play an active role in managing their treatments.

Incorporating biofilm-related treatments into clinical guidelines and best practice recommendations is another key strategy. By updating treatment protocols to include biofilm-specific interventions, healthcare institutions can ensure that practitioners have clear and evidence-based directives to follow.

Investing in technology and infrastructure that support the diagnosis and treatment of biofilm-associated infections is also essential. Advanced imaging techniques, laboratory assays, and biofilm-resistant medical devices can enhance the ability of healthcare providers to effectively manage these infections.

Furthermore, healthcare institutions can advocate for and participate in clinical trials evaluating biofilm-related treatments. By contributing to the body of evidence supporting these therapies, institutions can help accelerate their approval and integration into standard care practices.

Engaging with regulatory bodies and professional organizations is also important for promoting the adoption of biofilm-related treatments. These entities can provide the necessary frameworks and guidelines to ensure the safe and effective use of new therapies.

Healthcare institutions should also consider the economic aspects of biofilm-related treatments. By conducting cost-benefit analyses and working with insurance providers, they can help make these treatments more accessible to patients.

Lastly, institutions can leverage the power of data analytics to monitor the effectiveness of biofilm-related treatments and identify areas for improvement. By continuously evaluating treatment outcomes, healthcare providers can refine their approaches and optimize patient care.

In summary, the promotion of biofilm-related treatments in healthcare institutions requires a comprehensive and proactive approach that encompasses collaboration, education, integration into clinical practice, investment in technology, participation in research, engagement with regulatory bodies, economic considerations, and data-driven evaluation. These strategies can collectively enhance the adoption and effectiveness of biofilm-related treatments, ultimately leading to better patient outcomes and a reduction in the burden of biofilm-associated infections.

Patient advocacy groups (PAGs) play a pivotal role in the healthcare ecosystem, particularly in promoting treatments for complex conditions such as those involving biofilms. These groups serve as a bridge between patients, healthcare providers, researchers, and policymakers, ensuring that the voices and needs of patients are heard and addressed. PAGs can drive awareness about the importance of biofilm-related treatments and the challenges they address, such as antibiotic resistance and chronic infections. By leveraging their collective voice, PAGs have the power to influence research priorities and funding, advocating for the development of new treatments that target biofilms effectively.

Moreover, PAGs often participate in the regulatory process, providing testimony and patient perspectives that can shape the approval and adoption of new therapies. They work closely with researchers to identify unmet needs and potential therapeutic targets, and they can support clinical trials by helping to recruit participants and by disseminating information about the trials to their communities. PAGs also play a crucial role in education, not only for patients and their families but also for healthcare professionals who may not be fully aware of the latest developments in biofilm research and treatment.

In addition to these efforts, PAGs can influence policy at both the national and international levels, advocating for legislation that supports research and the approval of new treatments. They can also help to ensure that once treatments are approved, they are accessible to patients who need them, working with insurance companies and healthcare systems to include these treatments in coverage plans.

Furthermore, PAGs contribute to the scientific community by participating in conferences and publishing in scientific journals, sharing patient experiences and outcomes that can guide future research. They may also fundraise to support research directly or provide grants to scientists working on biofilm-related projects.

The role of PAGs is not limited to advocacy and education; they also provide support and resources to patients dealing with biofilm-associated conditions. This support can take many forms, from offering counseling and advice to creating support networks where patients can share their experiences and learn from each other.

In summary, patient advocacy groups are essential in promoting biofilm-related treatments. Their multifaceted efforts in advocacy, education, policy influence, support, and direct participation in the scientific process are invaluable in advancing the understanding and treatment of biofilm-associated conditions. Through their dedicated work, PAGs help to bring about change that can lead to better health outcomes for patients worldwide.

Patient advocacy groups (PAGs) have been instrumental in advancing biofilm research and treatment through various initiatives. One such initiative is the promotion of awareness and education about chronic wound infections, which are often complicated by biofilms. PAGs have worked to highlight the importance of innovative treatments, such as antimicrobial peptides and photodynamic therapy, which have shown promise in overcoming the challenges posed by biofilms. They have also been active in supporting research into antibiofilm peptides, which are crucial in the fight against biofilm-related treatment failure. These peptides have the potential to disrupt biofilms and enhance the efficacy of existing antibiotics, and PAGs have been pivotal in advocating for their development and inclusion in clinical practice.

In addition to these efforts, PAGs have played a key role in fostering collaboration between researchers, healthcare providers, and patients. This has led to the development of more effective strategies for managing biofilm-associated infections, such as the use of targeted therapies that address the unique properties of biofilms. By bringing together diverse stakeholders, PAGs have helped to ensure that research findings are translated into practical treatments that can benefit patients directly.

Furthermore, PAGs have been involved in policy-making processes, advocating for increased funding and support for biofilm research. Their efforts have contributed to the establishment of guidelines and protocols for the treatment of biofilm-related conditions, ensuring that patients receive the most up-to-date and effective care possible.

The impact of PAGs extends to the regulatory landscape as well. They have engaged with regulatory bodies to streamline the approval process for new biofilm-targeting treatments, making them more accessible to patients in need. This has been particularly important in the context of antibiotic resistance, where new solutions are urgently required.

PAGs have also been successful in raising public awareness about the significance of biofilms in chronic infections and the need for specialized treatments. Through campaigns, educational materials, and events, they have increased the visibility of biofilm-related issues and encouraged public support for research and development efforts.

Moreover, PAGs have contributed to the scientific community by participating in conferences and publishing in scientific journals. By sharing patient experiences and outcomes, they provide valuable insights that can guide future research and improve treatment approaches.

In summary, PAG-led initiatives have been successful in several areas related to biofilm research and treatment. From promoting awareness and education to advocating for policy changes and regulatory improvements, PAGs have been at the forefront of efforts to improve patient's lives dealing with biofilm-associated conditions. Their continued involvement is essential for the ongoing advancement of biofilm research and the development of new and effective treatments.

Patients and their families can become integral to PAG-led initiatives in biofilm research by engaging in a range of activities designed to support and advance the cause. Initially, they can start by identifying and connecting with PAGs that focus on conditions affected by biofilms. These groups often have websites and social media platforms where individuals can sign up for newsletters, attend informational webinars, and participate in community discussions. By becoming members, patients and families can stay informed about the latest research, treatment options, and advocacy opportunities.

Active participation in fundraising events is another way to contribute, as these efforts provide crucial financial support for biofilm research and awareness campaigns. Moreover, volunteering time and skills can be just as valuable; many PAGs rely on volunteers for organizing events, managing campaigns, and providing support to other patients and families.

Sharing personal stories and experiences with biofilm-related conditions is a powerful tool for advocacy. These narratives can be used in educational materials, presented at conferences, or shared with policymakers to highlight the real-world impact of biofilms on patients' lives. Such testimonials can drive home the urgency of advancing biofilm research and the development of new treatments.

Engagement in research efforts is also possible, with some PAGs facilitating connections between patients and research institutions. Patients and families can participate in clinical trials or observational studies, which are essential for developing new therapies and understanding the effectiveness of existing treatments.

Advocacy work is a critical component of PAG initiatives. Patients and families can advocate for increased funding, better policies, and greater public awareness by writing to legislators, participating in advocacy days, and joining campaigns that call for action on biofilm-related issues.

Furthermore, attending conferences and educational workshops can provide patients and families with deeper insights into biofilm research and treatments. These events are opportunities to learn from experts, ask questions, and network with other individuals who are navigating similar health challenges.

Patients and families can also support the creation and dissemination of educational content. By collaborating with PAGs, they can help develop brochures, videos, and online resources that inform and empower others affected by biofilm-associated conditions.

Lastly, providing feedback on treatment experiences and participating in surveys can help shape the direction of future research and healthcare practices. Patient-centered research is increasingly recognized as vital for ensuring that treatments meet the actual needs of those they are intended to help.

In summary, there are numerous ways for patients and their families to get involved with PAG-led initiatives in biofilm research. From raising awareness and funds to participating in advocacy and research, every contribution can make a significant difference in the fight against biofilm-related diseases.

For individuals grappling with biofilm-related conditions, finding support and community can be a significant aspect of managing their health. Online support groups offer a platform for patients to connect, share experiences, and access resources. While the search results indicate a variety of support groups for different health conditions, there are specific online communities that cater to patients dealing with biofilm-related issues. These groups often provide a space for individuals to discuss treatments, coping strategies, and the latest research. They may also offer educational materials and opportunities to participate in webinars or discussions with healthcare professionals. Additionally, some patient advocacy groups and foundations related to specific conditions associated with biofilms may host virtual support groups, offering regular meetings through video conferencing platforms where patients can join from the comfort of their homes. Registration for these groups is typically free, and they aim to create a safe and supportive environment for sharing and learning. It's important for patients and their families to engage with these groups as they can be a source of emotional support and practical advice, helping to navigate the complexities of biofilm-related conditions.

Green Chemistry Expansion:

Researchers are accelerating the development of environmentally friendly chemical processes. Green chemistry aims to minimize waste, reduce hazardous materials, and promote sustainable practices in drug discovery and manufacturing.

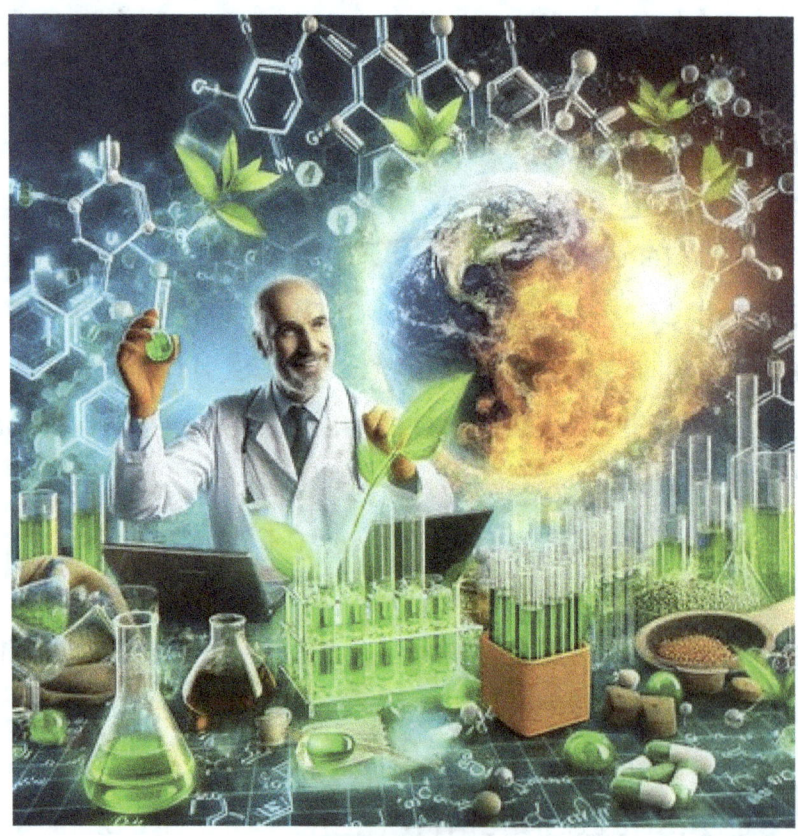

Green chemistry represents a transformative approach to the chemical sciences that emphasizes the design of products and processes that minimize or eliminate the use and generation of hazardous substances. This field is rapidly expanding as researchers and industries recognize the need to develop more sustainable practices in response to environmental concerns and resource limitations. The core of green chemistry lies in its twelve principles, which guide chemists in creating more environmentally benign substances and processes. These principles advocate for the use of safer chemicals, the design of energy-efficient processes, and the reduction of waste, among other sustainable practices.

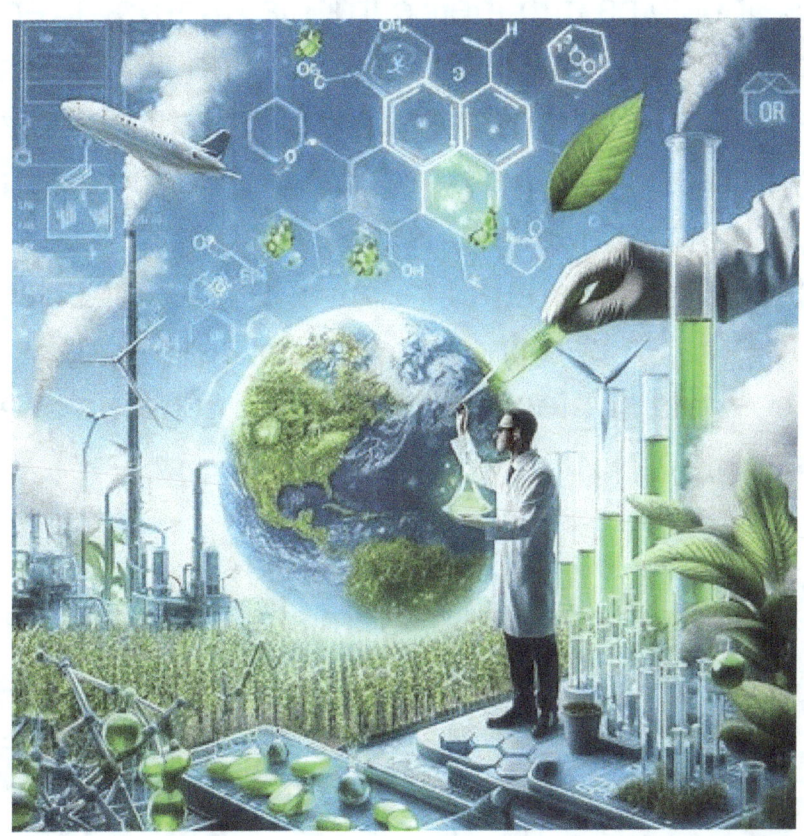

The expansion of green chemistry is evident in various sectors, including pharmaceuticals, where there is a significant push to develop drugs that are not only effective but also produced through environmentally friendly methods. This involves minimizing the use of toxic solvents and reagents, maximizing the efficiency of reactions, and designing degradation pathways for drugs to prevent environmental contamination. In manufacturing, green chemistry principles are being applied to reduce the environmental footprint of production processes. This includes the use of renewable feedstocks, the development of biodegradable materials, and the implementation of recycling and waste management strategies.

Educational institutions are also embracing green chemistry by incorporating its principles into their curricula, thereby preparing the next generation of chemists to think sustainably from the outset of their careers. Organizations like Beyond Benign are leading the way in green chemistry education, advocating for a systemic change in how chemistry is taught and practiced. The Green Chemistry Commitment, an initiative by Beyond Benign, has been instrumental in bringing together educational institutions to share resources and strategies for integrating green chemistry into their programs.

The industrial applications of green chemistry are becoming increasingly diverse, with companies exploring sustainable alternatives to traditional chemical processes. For example, the use of green solvents and the development of recyclable catalysts are becoming more prevalent in chemical synthesis. Energy efficiency is another area of focus, with industries seeking ways to reduce the energy consumption of chemical reactions, thereby lowering greenhouse gas emissions and operational costs.

The expansion of green chemistry is not without its challenges. One of the main hurdles is the need for full validation of chemical greenness by metrics that can accurately assess the environmental impact of chemical processes and products. Additionally, there is a need for increased collaboration between academia and industry to ensure that the research and development of green chemistry are aligned with practical applications.

Despite these challenges, the trend towards green chemistry is clear, with research showing a consistent increase in studies related to sustainable practices. The COVID-19 pandemic has slightly impacted the momentum, but the overall trajectory remains positive, indicating a growing commitment to environmental stewardship within the chemical sciences. As green chemistry continues to evolve, it holds the promise of a more sustainable future, where chemical innovations are in harmony with the health of our planet and its inhabitants.

Green chemistry is revolutionizing the field of drug discovery by introducing more sustainable and environmentally friendly methods. One notable example is Pfizer's approach to medicine development, where they focus on selecting materials that have less environmental impact, reducing resource use, minimizing waste, and running safe processes. They have also invested in continuous process technologies, which have led to significant reductions in waste and improvements in productivity.

Another example is the work done by Merck in developing a greener synthesis pathway for molnupiravir, an antiviral medication used to treat COVID-19. This new method reduced solvent waste, increased yield, and simplified the process from five steps to three, which was recognized with the Greener Reaction Conditions Award by the U.S. Environmental Protection Agency.

In academia, the book "Green Chemistry in Drug Discovery: From Academia to Industry" provides insights into the implementation of green chemistry in medicinal chemistry drug discovery. It covers a range of topics from greener approaches to chemical transformations that are prevalent in the pharmaceutical industry to the impact of enabling technologies in medicinal chemistry.

The adoption of green solvents and the development of recyclable catalysts are also becoming more common in chemical synthesis. For instance, the use of ionic liquids as green solvents has been explored for their potential to improve the sustainability of chemical reactions involved in drug synthesis.

Moreover, companies like Abbott, the Merck Group, Roche, Johnson and Johnson, Amgen, and Eli Lilly are making sincere efforts to utilize green chemistry processes throughout drug discovery, development, and manufacturing. These efforts include the use of non-toxic solvents and reagents, and the implementation of waste minimization strategies.

The advancement of green chemistry in drug discovery is not just limited to the use of safer chemicals and processes but also extends to the design of drugs themselves. Researchers are exploring synthetic routes to develop bioactive compounds, key intermediates, or pharmacophoric scaffolds with good atom economy and low carbon footprint. They are also investigating transformations in green solvents or no solvents at all, and the application of ultrasound for drug synthesis, which can lead to more efficient and less energy-intensive processes.

These examples illustrate the diverse ways in which green chemistry principles are being integrated into drug discovery and development. The shift towards more sustainable practices is a response to the growing awareness of the environmental impacts of pharmaceuticals and the need for the industry to adapt to a changing world. As green chemistry continues to evolve, it promises to play a crucial role in shaping a more sustainable future for the pharmaceutical industry and healthcare.

To delve deeper into the realm of green chemistry in drug discovery, a multifaceted approach to learning is beneficial. Engaging with comprehensive resources such as the book "Green Chemistry in Drug Discovery: From Academia to Industry" can provide a solid foundation in both the theoretical and practical aspects of green chemistry applications in the pharmaceutical sector. This book is particularly valuable as it offers insights from experts in the field and covers a range of topics from greener chemical transformations to the impact of enabling technologies in medicinal chemistry.

Additionally, exploring online platforms and databases for academic papers and industry reports can be incredibly informative. Websites like PubMed and ScienceDirect are repositories of numerous research articles where you can find the latest studies and reviews on green chemistry practices in drug development. Attending webinars, workshops, and conferences dedicated to green chemistry also presents an opportunity to learn from and network with professionals and researchers who are actively involved in this field.

Another avenue for learning is through educational courses offered by universities and online learning platforms. Many institutions now offer specialized courses in green chemistry and sustainable pharmaceutical practices, which can range from introductory to advanced levels. Online platforms like Coursera, edX, and Future Learn may provide courses that are accessible to a wider audience and can be taken at your own pace.

For a more hands-on experience, seeking internships or collaborative projects with laboratories and companies that are known for their green chemistry initiatives can be incredibly beneficial. Companies like Pfizer have been recognized for their sustainable approaches to medicine development and often share their knowledge and practices through various initiatives and publications.

Furthermore, joining professional organizations such as the American Chemical Society (ACS) and its Green Chemistry Institute can provide access to a wealth of resources, including publications, networking events, and educational materials. The ACS regularly hosts events and provides updates on the latest advancements in green chemistry.

Lastly, following industry news and subscribing to journals such as Green Chemistry, published by the Royal Society of Chemistry, can keep you informed about the latest trends and innovations in the field. Staying updated with the work of regulatory bodies like the U.S. Environmental Protection Agency (EPA), which defines and promotes green chemistry practices, is also crucial for understanding the broader impact and regulatory framework of green chemistry in drug discovery.

By combining these resources and opportunities for learning, you can build a comprehensive understanding of green chemistry principles and their application in drug discovery, paving the way for a more sustainable future in pharmaceuticals.

The key principles of green chemistry are foundational guidelines that aim to make chemical processes more sustainable and environmentally friendly. Developed by Paul Anastas and John Warner, these principles serve as a framework for chemists to design safer products and processes. The first principle is the prevention of waste, which emphasizes the importance of avoiding waste creation rather than treating or cleaning it up after its formation. Atom economy is another crucial principle, advocating for the design of methods that maximize the incorporation of all materials used in the process into the final product.

Less hazardous chemical syntheses are encouraged, where methods should be designed to use and generate substances with minimal toxicity to human health and the environment. In line with this, the design of safer chemicals is a principle that pushes for the creation of products that achieve their desired function while minimizing their toxicity. The use of safer solvents and auxiliaries is also promoted, aiming to eliminate the need for these substances or to ensure they are non-toxic when used.

Energy efficiency is a significant aspect of green chemistry, with the design of chemical processes that minimize energy consumption, ideally allowing for reactions to occur at ambient temperature and pressure. The use of renewable feedstocks is another principle, which involves utilizing materials that are renewable rather than depleting, whenever technically and economically viable.

Reducing derivatives is a principle that focuses on minimizing or avoiding unnecessary derivatization, which often requires additional reagents and can generate waste. Catalysis is favored over stoichiometric reagents, with the use of catalytic reagents that are as selective as possible being superior. The design for degradation principle ensures that chemical products are designed to break down into innocuous substances at the end of their functional life, preventing environmental persistence.

Real-time analysis for pollution prevention is a principle that calls for the development of analytical methodologies that allow for in-process monitoring and control to prevent the formation of hazardous substances. Lastly, inherently safer chemistry for accident prevention is a principle that selects substances and their forms to minimize the potential for chemical accidents, including releases, explosions, and fires.

These twelve principles of green chemistry are not just theoretical concepts but are actively being applied in research and industry to create a more sustainable future. They guide chemists and engineers in their efforts to innovate and transform the chemical landscape, ensuring that the products and processes they develop are in harmony with the environment. By adhering to these principles, the field of chemistry can significantly reduce its environmental footprint and contribute to the well-being of the planet and its inhabitants.

Clinical Validation of CRISPR:

CRISPR gene editing technology continues to evolve. In 2024, we'll likely see more clinical trials and applications of CRISPR-based therapies for various genetic disorders.

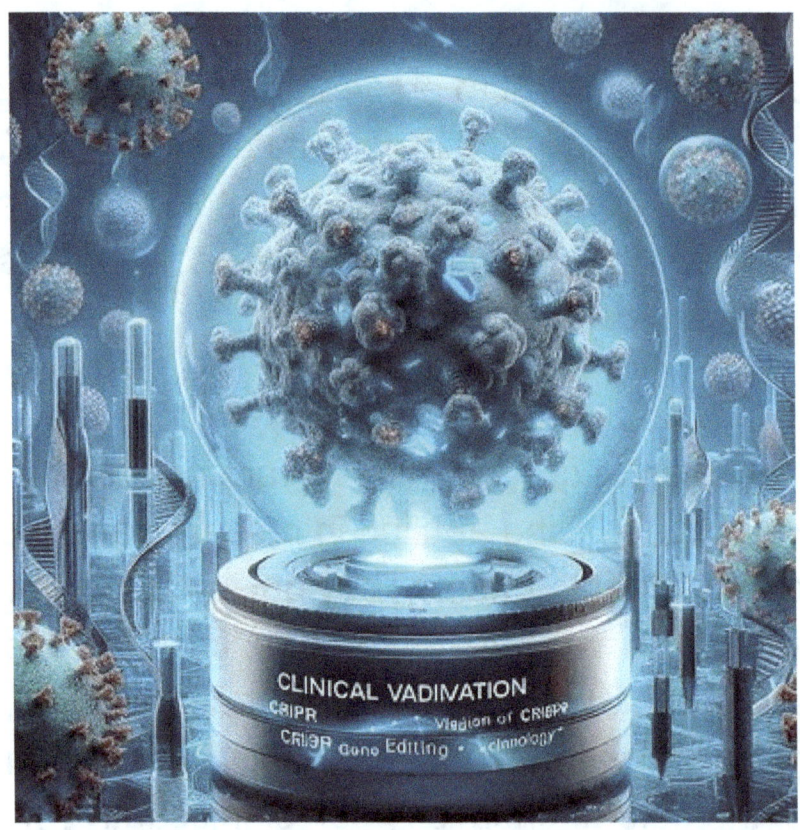

CRISPR (Clustered Regularly Interspaced Short Palindromic Repeats) gene editing technology has revolutionized the field of genetics, offering unprecedented precision in modifying DNA. The clinical validation of CRISPR has been a pivotal aspect of its development, ensuring that the technology is safe and effective for use in human medicine. As of 2024, the landscape of CRISPR-based therapies has expanded significantly, with the first-ever approval of a CRISPR-based medicine, Casgevy, marking a historic milestone in the treatment of genetic disorders such as sickle cell disease (SCD) and transfusion-dependent beta thalassemia (TDT).

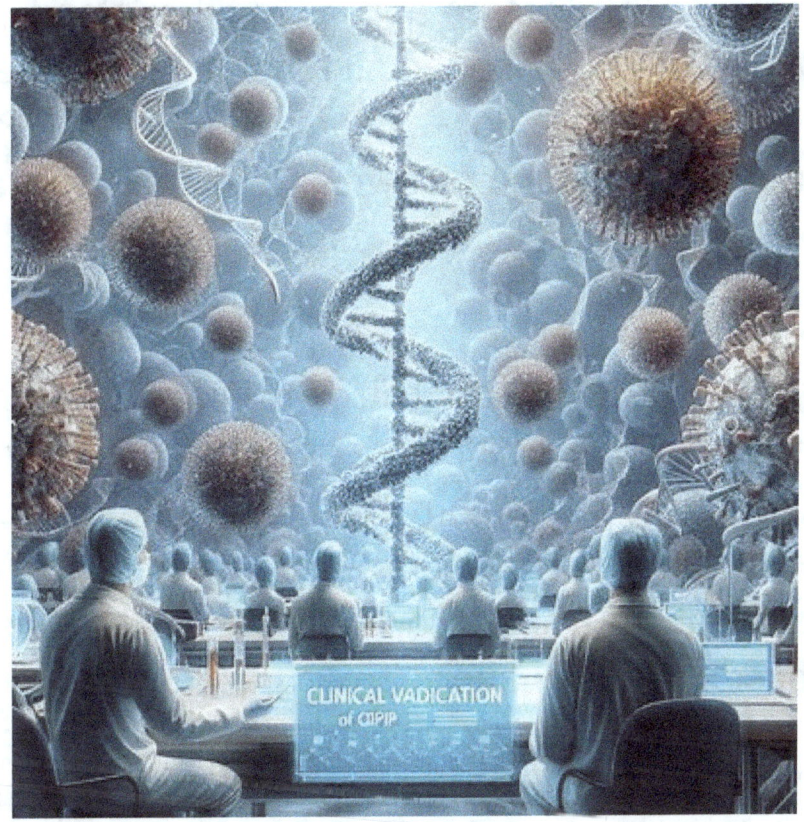

The approval of Casgevy by regulatory agencies like the UK's Medicines and Healthcare Products Regulatory Agency and the US Food and Drug Administration has set a precedent for the potential of CRISPR-based therapies. This has led to a surge in clinical trials aiming to explore the efficacy of CRISPR in treating a wide array of genetic conditions. The Innovative Genomics Institute (IGI) has been at the forefront of tracking the progress of these trials, highlighting the rapid advancement from laboratory research to approved therapies.

CRISPR's ability to induce the expression of fetal hemoglobin (HbF) in adults has been a game-changer for patients with SCD and TDT, as it compensates for the defective adult hemoglobin that these individuals lack. The success of these therapies has opened the door for CRISPR to be applied to other blood disorders, as well as diseases beyond the hematologic spectrum. For instance, clinical trials are now exploring the use of CRISPR for the treatment of autoimmune diseases, with the potential to significantly alter the therapeutic landscape.

The enthusiasm for CRISPR's capabilities is tempered by real-world challenges, such as the high cost of clinical trials and market forces that influence investment in biotechnology. Despite these hurdles, the field remains optimistic about the future of CRISPR-based therapies. The narrowing focus on the most developed products, due to financial pressures, has not dampened the spirit of innovation within the CRISPR community. Instead, it has led to a more targeted approach in advancing therapies that show the most promise.

Looking ahead, the potential applications of CRISPR are vast. Beyond treating genetic disorders, CRISPR technology is being explored for its utility in cancer precision medicine, where it can disrupt oncogenic targets and modulate the tumor microenvironment to enhance the efficacy of existing treatments. Additionally, CRISPR 2.0, a more refined version of the technology, is being tested in clinical trials for certain cancers and is expected to initiate trials for systemic lupus erythematosus and hematologic malignancies in the first half of 2024.

The clinical validation of CRISPR is not just about proving its therapeutic efficacy but also about addressing the ethical concerns that come with such a powerful tool. As CRISPR continues to evolve, it is imperative that its development is guided by rigorous ethical standards to ensure that its applications are beneficial and equitable. The journey of CRISPR from a novel scientific discovery to a validated clinical tool is a testament to the collaborative efforts of researchers, clinicians, and ethicists who are committed to harnessing its potential for the greater good.

In conclusion, the clinical validation of CRISPR in 2024 represents a significant leap forward in the field of gene editing. With the first CRISPR-based therapy approved and many more in the pipeline, the future of genetic medicine is poised for transformation. As CRISPR technologies continue to advance, they hold the promise of curing previously untreatable genetic diseases, enhancing our understanding of genetics, and opening new avenues for medical research and treatment.

CRISPR technology, while a groundbreaking tool in genetic engineering, carries several potential risks that are important to consider. One of the primary concerns is the possibility of "off-target" effects, where the CRISPR system may inadvertently alter DNA sequences similar to the target sequence, but which are not intended to be modified. This could potentially lead to unintended genetic mutations with unknown consequences. Another risk involves the delivery method of the CRISPR components into the cells; if not done correctly, it could lead to a low efficiency of gene editing or affect the survival of the cells.

Furthermore, there is a risk that CRISPR-edited cells might lose their ability to fight off cancers. Studies have suggested that the process of editing genes could inadvertently disable or weaken the function of tumor suppressor genes, thereby increasing the risk of cancer in those cells. Additionally, the long-term effects of gene editing are still not fully understood, and there is a concern that CRISPR might cause more damage to the genes than previously anticipated, which could have serious implications for the patient's health.

The ethical implications of CRISPR also pose a significant risk. The technology could potentially be used for non-therapeutic genetic modifications, such as creating "designer babies" with selected traits, which raises serious moral and ethical questions about the extent to which humans should interfere with natural genetic processes. There is also the issue of accessibility and equity; the high cost of CRISPR therapies could exacerbate existing inequalities in healthcare access and lead to a situation where only the wealthy can afford these life-altering treatments.

Moreover, the regulatory landscape for CRISPR is still evolving, and there may be risks associated with the lack of comprehensive legal and ethical guidelines to govern the use of this technology. Without clear regulations, there could be a gap in oversight, potentially leading to misuse or abuse of the technology.

In conclusion, while CRISPR has the potential to bring about significant medical advancements, it is crucial to proceed with caution. Ongoing research, ethical debates, and the development of robust regulatory frameworks are essential to ensure that CRISPR is used responsibly and for the benefit of all. As the technology continues to develop, it will be important to monitor and address these risks to harness CRISPR's full potential while minimizing its potential harms.

To mitigate the risks of off-target effects in CRISPR gene editing, researchers employ a multifaceted approach. One of the primary strategies involves the careful design of single-guide RNAs (sgRNAs) to enhance their specificity for the target DNA sequence. This is often achieved through in silico prediction tools that model CRISPR-Cas cleavage specificity, allowing for the selection of sgRNAs with minimal off-target potential. Additionally, modifications to the Cas9 enzyme itself, such as engineering high-fidelity variants or using Cas9 nickases that create single-strand breaks instead of double-strand breaks, can reduce the likelihood of off-target mutations.

Another technique is the use of truncated guide RNAs, which are shorter than the standard 20 nucleotides and can provide greater specificity. Researchers also utilize paired nickases, where two sgRNAs guide Cas9 nickases to adjacent sites on opposite DNA strands, resulting in a double-strand break that is highly specific to the target location. This method significantly lowers the risk of off-target effects because both sgRNAs must find their respective targets for the editing to occur.

The delivery method of the CRISPR components into cells is also crucial. Ribonucleoprotein (RNP) delivery, where the Cas9 protein and sgRNA are directly delivered as a complex, can reduce the duration of Cas9 activity in the cell, thereby decreasing the chances of off-target editing. Additionally, advancements in detection methods for off-target mutations, such as whole-genome sequencing and CRISPR-based assays, enable researchers to screen for and quantify off-target effects more effectively.

Furthermore, the development of base editors, which are engineered proteins capable of making single nucleotide changes without creating double-strand breaks, offers a more precise editing option with reduced off-target risks. Prime editing, another recent innovation, allows for the direct writing of new genetic information into a specified DNA site without double-strand breaks or donor DNA templates, further minimizing unintended edits.

Ethical considerations are also paramount in mitigating risks. Researchers adhere to strict ethical guidelines and conduct thorough pre-clinical risk assessments to ensure the safety of CRISPR therapeutics. Regulatory bodies play a critical role in this process, setting standards and approving therapies only after rigorous evaluation of their safety and efficacy.

In summary, the mitigation of off-target effects in CRISPR gene editing is a dynamic field that combines advanced molecular biology techniques, computational tools, and ethical oversight.

Through these concerted efforts, researchers aim to harness the full potential of CRISPR while ensuring the highest standards of safety for future therapeutic applications.

Current off-target prediction tools for CRISPR gene editing are essential for identifying potential unintended edits in the genome. However, these tools have limitations that can impact their accuracy and reliability. One significant limitation is that many prediction tools may not fully account for the complexity of the genome, such as its three-dimensional structure and epigenetic factors, which can influence the binding of the CRISPR-Cas9 complex to the DNA. Additionally, the predictive models often rely on in vitro or in silico data, which may not perfectly translate to in vivo conditions where the cellular environment can affect the outcome of gene editing.

Another challenge is the limited understanding of the CRISPR-Cas9 molecular mechanism, which hinders the ability of computational tools to predict off-target effects with high confidence. The tools may also struggle with the precision-recall trade-off, where increasing the sensitivity to detect potential off-target sites can lead to a higher false-positive rate, making it difficult to discern true off-target events from background noise. Furthermore, some tools may have restrictive sets of parameters, take too few mismatches into account for off-target search, or lack full documentation about potential off-target sites, which can limit their effectiveness.

The current tools also vary in their ability to predict off-target effects in different genomic contexts, such as those with high GC content or low complexity regions, which are more prone to off-target cleavage. This variability can lead to inconsistencies in off-target predictions across different tools, making it challenging for researchers to reach a consensus on the safety of a particular CRISPR edit. Moreover, the tools may not always be user-friendly, with some requiring extensive bioinformatics expertise to interpret the results accurately.

To address these limitations, ongoing research is focused on improving the algorithms and incorporating more comprehensive genomic data into the prediction models. Advances in machine learning and artificial intelligence are being leveraged to enhance the predictive power of these tools, allowing for more accurate and reliable off-target effect predictions. Additionally, the development of new experimental methods to validate the predictions in vivo is crucial for confirming the safety and efficacy of CRISPR-based therapies.

In summary, while off-target prediction tools are invaluable for the safe application of CRISPR gene editing, they are not without their limitations. Researchers must be aware of these constraints and continue to refine the tools and validation methods to ensure the responsible use of CRISPR technology in clinical and research settings. As the field progresses, it is expected that the prediction and mitigation of off-target effects will become increasingly precise, paving the way for safer and more effective gene editing therapies.

How does CRISPR work at a molecular level?

CRISPR-Cas9 operates at a molecular level as a highly sophisticated and precise method of genetic editing. The system originates from a natural defense mechanism found in bacteria and archaea, providing immunity against invading viruses. The core components of CRISPR-Cas9 include the Cas9 enzyme, which acts as molecular scissors, and a piece of RNA known as guide RNA (gRNA). The gRNA is designed to match a specific DNA sequence in the genome that is targeted for editing. When introduced into a cell, the gRNA binds to the Cas9 enzyme, and this complex then navigates through the cell's nucleus to locate the target DNA sequence.

Upon finding the correct sequence, the gRNA binds to the DNA, and the Cas9 enzyme performs a precise cut across both strands of the DNA helix. This cut effectively disables the target gene, preventing it from functioning. Alternatively, the cell's natural DNA repair mechanisms can be harnessed to introduce changes to the gene. When the DNA is cut, the cell attempts to repair the break. Researchers can exploit this repair process by providing a piece of DNA with the desired sequence, which the cell can use as a template to repair the cut DNA. This allows for the addition of new genetic material or the correction of mutations.

The precision of CRISPR-Cas9 comes from the ability of the gRNA to bind only to the complementary DNA sequence, ensuring that cuts are made at specific locations. However, the system is not infallible; sometimes, the Cas9 enzyme can bind to and cut sequences that are similar but not identical to the target sequence, leading to off-target effects. These unintended edits are a significant concern for the application of CRISPR-Cas9 in therapeutic settings, where precision is crucial.

To enhance the specificity of CRISPR-Cas9, researchers have developed modified versions of the Cas9 enzyme and the gRNA. High-fidelity Cas9 variants have been engineered to reduce off-target activity, and changes to the gRNA structure can increase its binding specificity. Additionally, alternative CRISPR systems, such as Cas12 and Cas13, offer different mechanisms of action and can target RNA as well as DNA, expanding the potential applications of CRISPR technology.

The molecular mechanism of CRISPR-Cas9 has opened up vast possibilities in genetic research and medicine. It has the potential to treat genetic disorders, create disease-resistant crops, and even eradicate infectious diseases by targeting the genetic material of pathogens. As research progresses, the CRISPR-Cas9 system continues to evolve, with improvements in its efficiency, specificity, and versatility, making it one of the most powerful tools in modern biology.

The guide RNA (gRNA) within the CRISPR-Cas9 system is a fundamental component that drives the specificity of the gene editing process. It is designed to recognize and bind to a complementary DNA sequence in the genome, which is targeted for editing. The gRNA is composed of two key parts: the CRISPR RNA (crRNA) and the trans-activating crRNA (tracrRNA). The crRNA contains a 17-20 nucleotide sequence that is complementary to the target DNA sequence, and this allows it to act as a homing device, guiding the Cas9 enzyme to the precise location where an edit is intended.

The tracrRNA portion serves as a binding scaffold for the Cas9 nuclease, facilitating the formation of a complex between the gRNA and Cas9. This complex then searches the cell's DNA for a match to the crRNA's sequence. Once the target DNA sequence is found, the gRNA/Cas9 complex binds to it, positioning the Cas9 to make a cut at the specified location. The specificity of this interaction is further enhanced by the requirement for a Protospacer Adjacent Motif (PAM) sequence, which is a short, conserved sequence following the target DNA sequence that is essential for Cas9 binding and cleavage.

The PAM sequence recognition is a critical aspect of the targeting process because it provides a double-check mechanism, ensuring that the Cas9 enzyme does not bind to and cut random sites throughout the genome. The PAM sequence is recognized by the Cas9 protein, not the gRNA, which adds an extra layer of specificity to the system. Different types of Cas proteins require different PAM sequences, and this requirement must be considered when designing gRNAs for gene editing experiments.

The design of the gRNA is a crucial step in the CRISPR process, as it needs to be highly specific to the target sequence to avoid off-target effects. Computational tools and databases of validated gRNA sequences are available to assist researchers in designing gRNAs that maximize on-target activity while minimizing potential off-target effects. These tools consider various factors, such as the genomic context of the target site and the presence of similar sequences elsewhere in the genome that could lead to off-target binding and cleavage.

Despite the high specificity of gRNA targeting, off-target effects can still occur, which is why researchers often employ multiple methods to predict and verify the precision of gRNA targeting. These methods include in silico prediction tools, in vitro cleavage assays, and in vivo validation experiments. The ongoing development of more sophisticated gRNA design algorithms and the refinement of Cas enzymes for improved specificity are active areas of research aimed at enhancing the safety and efficacy of CRISPR-Cas9 gene editing.

In summary, the gRNA recognizes its target sequence through a combination of complementary base pairing between the crRNA and the target DNA, the presence of a PAM sequence, and the formation of a complex with the Cas9 enzyme. The precision of this system is the result of a delicate interplay between the gRNA design, the Cas9 enzyme's properties, and the genomic context of the target sequence. As the field of gene editing advances, the mechanisms of gRNA targeting continue to be refined, ensuring that CRISPR technology remains a powerful and precise tool for genetic manipulation.

Optimizing guide RNA (gRNA) design is a critical step in ensuring the success of CRISPR-Cas9 gene editing applications. Researchers tailor gRNA sequences to maximize efficiency and specificity for their experimental needs. The optimization process begins with the selection of the target DNA sequence. This sequence must be unique to the region of interest to avoid off-target effects, and it must be adjacent to a Protospacer Adjacent Motif (PAM), which is essential for Cas9 binding and cleavage.

Once the target sequence is identified, researchers use computational tools to predict the efficiency and specificity of potential gRNAs. These tools assess factors such as the gRNA's binding energy, the likelihood of off-target binding, and the presence of secondary structures that could impede the gRNA's interaction with the target DNA. Advances in machine learning and deep learning have led to the development of more sophisticated prediction models that can more accurately forecast gRNA performance.

In addition to computational predictions, empirical testing is crucial. Researchers often synthesize several candidate gRNAs and test them in cell lines or model organisms to observe their editing efficiency and potential off-target effects. High-throughput screening methods allow for the simultaneous assessment of multiple gRNA candidates, streamlining the selection process.

Modifications to the gRNA structure can also enhance its function. For example, chemical modifications such as 2'-O-methyl analogs and phosphorothioate backbones can increase gRNA stability and resistance to nucleases, thereby improving its lifespan and effectiveness within the cell. Truncated gRNAs, which are shorter than the standard 20 nucleotides, have been shown to reduce off-target activity while maintaining on-target efficiency.

The delivery method of the gRNA-Cas9 complex into cells is another area of optimization. Researchers choose between methods such as plasmid, viral, or ribonucleoprotein (RNP) delivery based on the specific requirements of their study. RNP delivery, for instance, offers a transient expression of the Cas9-gRNA complex, reducing the duration of Cas9 activity in the cell and thus the potential for off-target effects.

For applications requiring high precision, such as therapeutic gene editing, researchers may employ Cas9 variants with enhanced specificity. These high-fidelity Cas9 enzymes have been engineered to reduce off-target cleavage without compromising on-target activity. Additionally, alternative CRISPR systems like Cas12 and Cas13 provide different PAM requirements and targeting capabilities, expanding the toolbox available for gRNA design.

Ethical considerations also play a role in gRNA optimization. For clinical applications, the safety profile of the gRNA-Cas9 system is paramount. Researchers must ensure that their gRNA designs minimize the risk of unintended genetic modifications that could have adverse effects. Regulatory guidelines often influence the design process, as gRNA sequences must meet safety standards set by bodies such as the FDA or EMA.

In summary, optimizing gRNA design for specific applications is a multifaceted process that involves careful target selection, computational predictions, empirical validation, structural modifications, delivery method considerations, and ethical compliance. The goal is to create a gRNA that is highly efficient, specific to the target site, stable within the cell, and safe for use in the intended application. As CRISPR technology continues to evolve, so will the strategies for gRNA optimization, enabling more precise and effective gene editing across a wide range of research and clinical contexts.

Optimizing guide RNA (gRNA) design for therapeutic applications presents several challenges that researchers must navigate to ensure safety and efficacy. One of the primary challenges is achieving high specificity to minimize off-target effects, which can lead to unintended genetic alterations and potential adverse effects. The complexity of the human genome, with its repetitive sequences and structural variations, makes it difficult to design gRNAs that exclusively target the intended site without interacting with similar sequences elsewhere in the genome.

Another significant challenge is the delivery of the gRNA-Cas9 complex to the target cells in the body. Effective delivery must ensure that the complex reaches the desired cells in sufficient quantities, without eliciting an immune response or causing toxicity. This is particularly challenging when targeting tissues that are hard to reach or protected by biological barriers, such as the brain or the inner ear.

The stability of the gRNA within the cellular environment is also a concern. gRNAs are susceptible to degradation by cellular nucleases, which can reduce their effectiveness. Chemical modifications can increase stability, but these must be balanced against the potential impact on gRNA binding and Cas9 activity.

In addition to these technical challenges, there are also ethical and regulatory hurdles. The possibility of germline editing raises ethical questions about the long-term implications and potential for heritable changes. Regulatory bodies are still developing frameworks to evaluate the safety and ethical considerations of gRNA therapies, which can slow down the translation from research to clinical application.

Furthermore, the cost of developing gRNA therapies can be prohibitive, limiting access to these treatments. The need for individualized gRNA design for each patient or condition adds to the complexity and cost, making it challenging to develop broadly applicable solutions.

Researchers are addressing these challenges through various strategies, such as improving computational tools for gRNA design, developing more efficient delivery vectors, and conducting rigorous preclinical studies to assess safety and efficacy. Advances in nanotechnology and the development of novel Cas enzymes with higher specificity are also contributing to overcoming these obstacles.

In conclusion, while the optimization of gRNA design for therapeutic applications holds great promise, it is a complex process fraught with scientific, ethical, and logistical challenges. Continued research and collaboration across disciplines are essential to address these challenges and realize the full therapeutic potential of CRISPR-Cas9 gene editing.

Enhancing the specificity of guide RNA (gRNA) in therapeutic applications is crucial to ensure that CRISPR-Cas9 gene editing is both safe and effective. Researchers have developed several strategies to achieve this goal. One approach is the engineering of Cas9 nuclease to create high-fidelity variants that reduce off-target effects. These variants are designed to be more selective in their DNA binding and cleavage, thereby increasing the precision of the gene editing process.

Another strategy involves the optimization of gRNA design. This includes adjusting the length and composition of the gRNA to improve its binding specificity to the target DNA sequence. Computational tools are often used to predict potential off-target sites and to design gRNAs that minimize these risks. Additionally, chemical modifications can be made to the gRNA to enhance its stability and reduce degradation by cellular nucleases, which can otherwise lead to reduced specificity.

The delivery method of the gRNA-Cas9 complex is also a key factor in enhancing specificity. Direct delivery methods, such as ribonucleoprotein (RNP) complexes, can provide a controlled and transient expression of the Cas9-gRNA complex, reducing the window of time during which off-target effects could occur. Moreover, the use of base editors and prime editors, which are newer technologies that allow for direct, single-base editing without creating double-strand breaks, can offer a more precise editing option with a lower risk of off-target effects.

Researchers also employ strategies to control the activity of Cas9, such as using inducible promoters or self-limiting circuits that regulate the expression of Cas9, thus minimizing the potential for off-target editing. Additionally, the use of anti-CRISPR proteins or CRISPR inhibitors can provide a means to fine-tune the activity of the Cas9 enzyme, further enhancing specificity.

In summary, the enhancement of gRNA specificity in therapeutic applications involves a combination of nuclease engineering, gRNA design optimization, careful selection of delivery methods, and control of Cas9 activity. These strategies are critical for advancing the therapeutic potential of CRISPR-Cas9 technology while maintaining the highest standards of safety and efficacy. As research in this field continues to evolve, it is likely that new and improved methods for increasing gRNA specificity will emerge, further refining the precision of gene editing therapies.

High-fidelity Cas9 variants and wild-type Cas9 are both derived from the CRISPR-Cas9 system, which is widely used for genome editing due to its precision and versatility. The key differences between these two forms of Cas9 primarily lie in their specificity and the likelihood of off-target effects, which are crucial considerations in therapeutic applications.

Wild-type Cas9, the original form of the enzyme derived from Streptococcus pyogenes, is highly efficient at cutting DNA at target sites specified by guide RNA (gRNA). However, it can also bind to and cleave sequences that are not perfectly matched to the gRNA, leading to off-target mutations. These unintended edits can have significant implications, especially in a clinical context where safety is paramount.

High-fidelity Cas9 variants, on the other hand, have been engineered to reduce these off-target effects. They are designed with specific mutations that weaken the non-specific interactions between the Cas9-gRNA complex and the DNA. This results in a more stringent requirement for base-pairing between the gRNA and the target DNA sequence, thereby enhancing the specificity of the gene editing process. For example, enhanced SpCas9 (eSpCas9(1.1)) and SpCas9-High Fidelity (SpCas9-HF1) are two such variants that have been developed to improve the precision of CRISPR-Cas9 editing.

The development of high-fidelity Cas9 variants involves detailed analysis of the Cas9 structure and its interaction with DNA. By understanding the molecular basis of off-target binding, researchers have been able to identify and introduce mutations that reduce this undesired activity. For instance, the eSpCas9(1.1) variant has been created through the hypothesis that certain amino acid substitutions could reduce off-target cleavage by weakening the interactions that do not contribute to specific DNA targeting.

Another high-fidelity variant, HypaCas9, was generated by analyzing crystal structures of Cas9 variants and identifying new mutations that could further enhance accuracy. These high-fidelity variants are valuable tools for genome editing, particularly in applications where precision is critical, such as in the development of gene therapies.

The high-fidelity Cas9 variants are not only more specific but also retain robust on-target activity. This means that while they are less likely to cause off-target effects, they are still highly effective at making the desired edits at the target sites. This balance between specificity and efficiency is a key advantage of high-fidelity Cas9 variants over the wild-type enzyme.

In addition to the engineered high-fidelity variants, there are also naturally occurring Cas9 proteins from different bacterial species that have different PAM requirements and targeting capabilities. These natural variants expand the range of potential target sites within the genome and can be selected based on the specific needs of the editing application.

Overall, the key differences between high-fidelity Cas9 variants and wild-type Cas9 hinge on their specificity and the risk of off-target effects. High-fidelity variants offer a safer and more precise alternative for genome editing, particularly in therapeutic contexts where the accuracy of gene editing is of utmost importance. As the field of genome editing continues to advance, the development and refinement of high-fidelity Cas9 variants will remain a critical area of research, with the potential to significantly impact the future of genetic medicine.

High-fidelity Cas9 variants are engineered forms of the Cas9 protein that have been modified to increase their specificity and reduce off-target effects, which are particularly important for therapeutic applications. These variants, such as eSpCas9(1.1) and SpCas9-HF1, have mutations that weaken non-specific interactions with DNA, thus requiring a more precise match between the guide RNA (gRNA) and the target DNA sequence.

In contrast, Cas12 (formerly known as Cpf1) is a different type of CRISPR system that has some distinct features when compared to Cas9. Cas12a, for example, requires a T-rich Protospacer Adjacent Motif (PAM) sequence and creates a 'staggered' cut in the DNA, which can be advantageous for certain applications, such as non-homologous end joining (NHEJ) or homology-directed repair (HDR). Cas12 enzymes are also capable of processing multiple crRNAs from a single transcript, which allows for multiplexed genome editing.

Cas13, on the other hand, is unique in that it targets RNA instead of DNA. This makes it particularly useful for applications that require transient modulation of gene expression, such as knockdown experiments or the study of RNA viruses. Cas13's mechanism involves two higher eukaryotes and prokaryotes nucleotide-binding (HEPN) domains that cleave RNA upon recognition of the target sequence.

When comparing high-fidelity Cas9 variants to Cas12 and Cas13, it's important to consider the specific requirements of the intended application. High-fidelity Cas9 variants are ideal for applications where DNA specificity is paramount, and the risk of off-target effects must be minimized. Cas12 may be preferred for its distinct PAM requirements and staggered cutting pattern, which can facilitate certain types of genome editing. Cas13's RNA-targeting capability opens up possibilities for controlling gene expression without altering the genome, which can be beneficial for therapeutic strategies that aim to manage, rather than cure, genetic diseases.

Each system has its own set of advantages and limitations. High-fidelity Cas9 variants, while more specific, may still carry a risk of off-target effects, albeit reduced. Cas12's requirement for a T-rich PAM sequence may limit its targeting range compared to Cas9. Cas13's RNA-targeting nature means it cannot be used for permanent genome editing, but it offers a safer profile for certain therapeutic applications where temporary modulation is desired.

In summary, high-fidelity Cas9 variants are designed to improve the specificity of DNA targeting, reducing the likelihood of off-target effects, which is crucial for therapeutic use. Cas12 and Cas13 offer alternative PAM requirements, cutting patterns, and target molecules (DNA vs. RNA), expanding the CRISPR toolkit and providing researchers with more options to tailor their genome editing approaches to the needs of their specific applications. The choice between these systems will depend on factors such as the type of edit required, the target site, and the desired outcome of the editing process. As the field of genome editing evolves, the development of new CRISPR systems and the refinement of existing ones will continue to enhance the precision and safety of gene editing technologies.

Rise of Biomaterials:

Biomaterials are essential for tissue engineering, drug delivery, and medical devices. Researchers are developing innovative materials that interact seamlessly with the human body, promoting healing and improving patient outcomes.

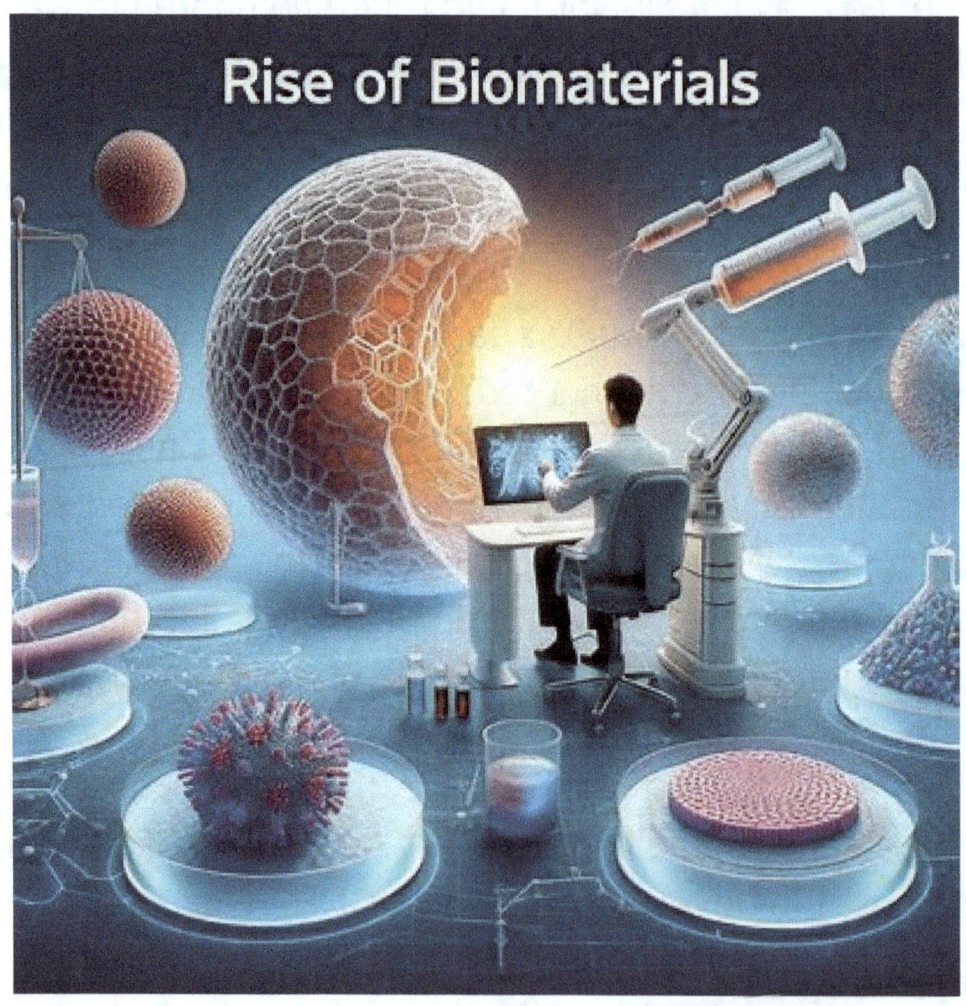

Biomaterials represent a revolutionary leap forward in the fields of tissue engineering, drug delivery, and the creation of medical devices. These materials are engineered to perform complex biological functions and are integral to the advancement of regenerative medicine. They are designed to interact with human tissues and systems without causing adverse reactions, making them indispensable for a wide range of medical applications.

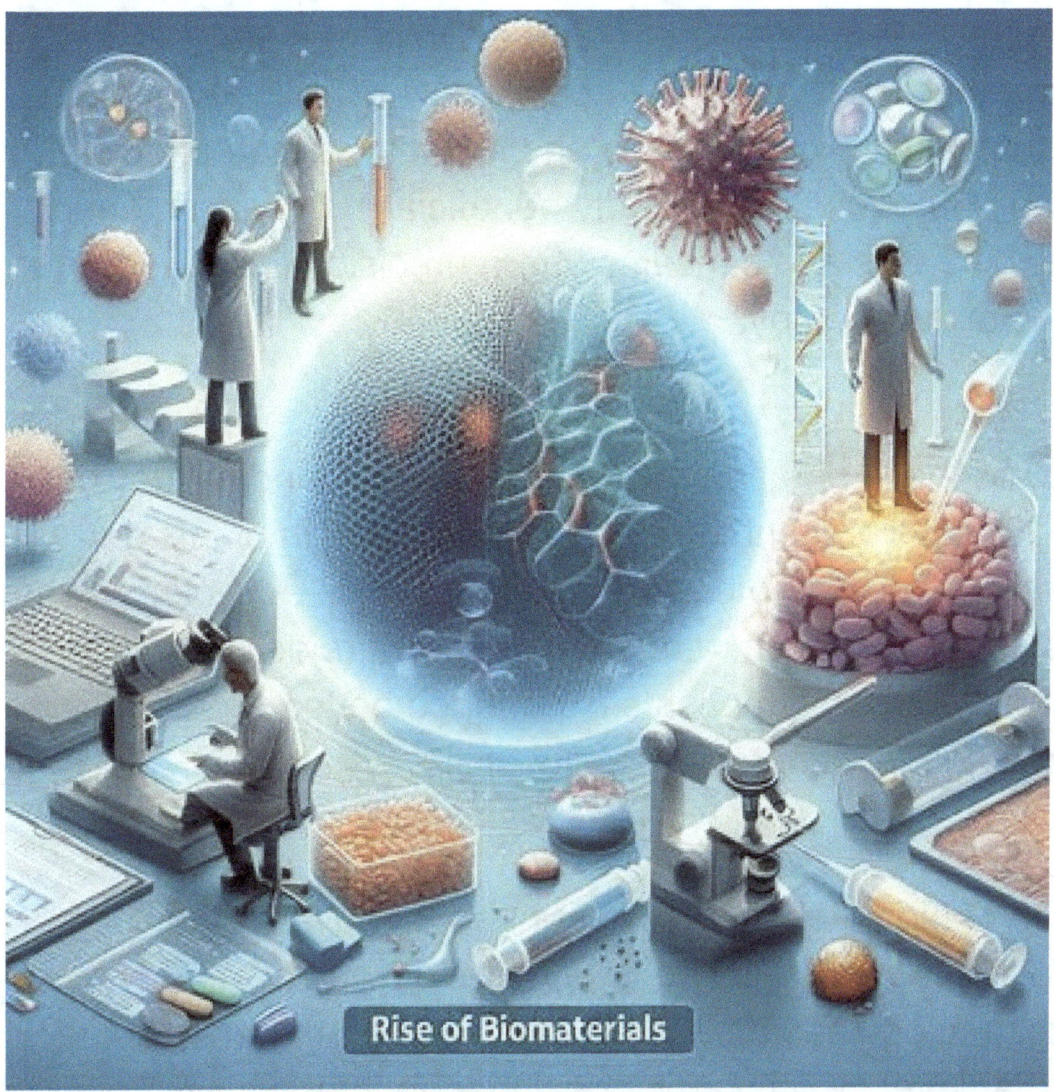

Rise of Biomaterials

In tissue engineering, biomaterials provide the scaffolding necessary to support the growth and regeneration of new tissues. This is crucial for repairing or replacing damaged organs and tissues, offering hope for patients with previously untreatable conditions. The versatility of biomaterials allows for the development of highly specialized scaffolds that can mimic the natural environment of cells, promoting proper cell function and integration into the body.

Drug delivery systems have also been transformed by the use of biomaterials. They enable targeted delivery of therapeutics, ensuring that drugs reach the specific site of action within the body, thus maximizing efficacy and minimizing side effects. This targeted approach is particularly beneficial in the treatment of chronic diseases and cancers, where precision is key to the success of the therapy.

Moreover, the integration of biomaterials into medical devices has led to the development of more biocompatible implants and prosthetics. These devices are designed to be accepted by the body's immune system, reducing the risk of rejection and infection. As a result, patients experience better long-term outcomes and an improved quality of life.

The rise of biomaterials is underpinned by advancements in nanotechnology, bioprinting, and materials science. Nanotechnology has enabled the creation of materials at the molecular level, which can be designed to interact with cells and tissues in highly specific ways. Bioprinting, on the other hand, utilizes biomaterials to create three-dimensional structures that closely resemble natural tissues, offering new possibilities for organ transplantation and repair.

The field of biomaterials is not without its challenges, however. The complexity of the human body means that creating materials that can reliably interact with it requires a deep understanding of biology, chemistry, and physics. Researchers must also navigate the ethical considerations and regulatory requirements associated with introducing new materials into the body.

Despite these challenges, the potential of biomaterials to improve patient outcomes is immense. As research continues to advance, we can expect to see even more innovative applications of biomaterials that will push the boundaries of what is possible in medicine and healthcare. The rise of biomaterials is a testament to the incredible progress being made at the intersection of biology and engineering, heralding a new era of medical treatments that are more effective, less invasive, and more personalized than ever before.

Biomaterials are a diverse group of materials that are engineered to safely interact with biological systems for medical purposes. Examples of biomaterials include metals like titanium and stainless steel, which are used in orthopedic implants such as hip replacements and bone plates due to their strength and biocompatibility. Ceramics, another category, are utilized for their durability and similarity to bone minerals; they are often found in dental implants and bone grafts. Polymers, both natural and synthetic, are widely used for their versatility and can be found in items such as contact lenses, heart valves, and artificial tendons.

Additionally, composites, which combine two or more different materials, are employed to take advantage of the unique properties of each component. For instance, carbon fiber-reinforced polymers are used in prosthetics for their lightweight and high-strength characteristics. Hydrogels, which can absorb large amounts of water, are used in wound dressings and drug delivery systems due to their biocompatibility and ability to release drugs over time.

Living cells and tissues are also considered biomaterials when used in medical applications. Engineered tissues and organs, grown in the lab using techniques like 3D bioprinting, are promising areas of research that could lead to personalized medicine solutions. Bioactive glasses and ceramics are designed to bond well with surrounding tissue and are used in applications such as bone regeneration.

The field of biomaterials is constantly evolving, with researchers developing new materials that can interact with the body in innovative ways. For example, smart biomaterials can respond to stimuli such as temperature or pH changes, making them useful in dynamic environments within the body. Nanomaterials, designed at the molecular level, offer precision in targeting diseased cells or tissues, opening new possibilities in cancer treatment and regenerative medicine.

The use of biomaterials is not limited to implants and tissue engineering; they also play a crucial role in diagnostic devices, biosensors, and drug delivery systems. For instance, biosensors made of biomaterials can detect specific substances in the body and provide critical information for disease management. Drug delivery systems utilizing biomaterials can control the release of medication, improving treatment efficacy and patient compliance.

In summary, biomaterials are integral to modern medicine, offering solutions that enhance the quality of life for patients around the world. Their development requires a multidisciplinary approach, combining knowledge from biology, chemistry, materials science, and engineering to create materials that are safe, effective, and tailored to meet the complex needs of human biology.

The future of biomaterials in medicine is poised to be transformative, with advancements that promise to redefine healthcare and patient outcomes. The ongoing research and development in this field is focusing on creating materials that are not only biocompatible but also capable of performing complex biological functions. One of the most exciting prospects is the development of protein-based materials for tissue engineering, which could provide scaffolds that support the growth and regeneration of tissues, potentially revolutionizing organ transplantation and repair.

Lipid-based materials are another area of significant interest, particularly for their potential in targeted drug delivery systems. These materials could enable medications to be delivered directly to the affected area, thereby increasing efficacy and reducing side effects. Bioelectronic materials are also on the horizon, offering the potential to integrate electronic functionality with biological systems, which could lead to breakthroughs in prosthetics and neural interfaces.

The innovation doesn't stop there; bioinks used in 3D bioprinting are advancing, allowing for the creation of more complex tissue structures. Self-healing materials that can repair themselves after damage are being developed, which could extend the lifespan of implants and reduce the need for replacement surgeries. Programmable materials that can change their properties in response to external stimuli are expected to open new possibilities in responsive drug delivery and dynamic tissue scaffolding.

Antibacterial materials are also a critical area of research, especially in the face of rising antimicrobial resistance. These materials could offer new ways to prevent and treat infections, particularly in hospital settings where infection control is paramount. Additionally, the push for sustainability in healthcare is leading to the development of sustainable materials, including biodegradable medical supplies, which could help reduce the environmental impact of medical waste.

The integration of advanced machine learning approaches with biomaterials research is enhancing the precision and personalization of medical treatments. This combination is expected to lead to more personalized medicine, where treatments and materials are tailored to the individual's specific biological makeup.

Nanotechnology continues to play a pivotal role in the future of biomaterials, enabling the design of materials at the molecular level for highly specific interactions with cells and tissues. This precision is particularly beneficial in the treatment of diseases like cancer, where targeted therapies can significantly improve patient outcomes.

The potential applications of biomaterials extend beyond traditional medical devices and implants. They are becoming increasingly important in diagnostic devices, biosensors, and even in the emerging field of biohybrid systems, where biological and synthetic components are combined to create new functionalities.

As the field of biomaterials progresses, it is also addressing the challenges of biocompatibility and immune response. Researchers are working to understand and mitigate the body's reaction to foreign materials, aiming to create biomaterials that are not only accepted by the body but also promote healing and integration.

In conclusion, the future of biomaterials in medicine is bright, with ongoing research paving the way for innovations that will enhance the quality of life for patients worldwide. The advancements in this field are set to provide solutions that are more effective, less invasive, and tailored to the individual needs of patients, marking a new era in medical science and healthcare delivery.

Developing biomaterials presents a myriad of challenges that span across scientific, technical, and ethical domains. One of the primary challenges is ensuring biocompatibility, which means the material must not elicit an adverse reaction from the body's immune system and should support cellular functions and tissue integration. Achieving this requires a deep understanding of the complex interactions between biomaterials and biological systems, which is still an area of ongoing research.

Another significant challenge is the degradation behavior of biomaterials. They must degrade at a rate that matches the tissue healing process to avoid inflammatory responses or toxicity due to the accumulation of degradation products. This necessitates precise control over the material's properties, which can be difficult to achieve consistently.

The mechanical properties of biomaterials also pose a challenge. They need to mimic the natural properties of the tissues they are replacing or supporting, which can vary widely. For example, materials used in bone tissue engineering must be strong and supportive, while those used in soft tissue applications require flexibility and elasticity.

Sterilization is another critical issue. Biomaterials must be sterilizable without losing their beneficial properties or becoming toxic. However, traditional sterilization methods can sometimes alter the physical and chemical properties of biomaterials, rendering them less effective or even harmful.

Furthermore, the scale-up from laboratory to clinical application is a significant hurdle. Materials that show promise in small-scale experiments often face unforeseen challenges when produced in larger quantities or when used in the complex environment of the human body.

Regulatory approval is also a lengthy and costly process. Biomaterials must undergo rigorous testing to meet safety and efficacy standards set by regulatory bodies like the FDA. This process can take many years and requires substantial investment, which can be a barrier to innovation and market entry.

Ethical considerations are also at play, particularly when it comes to materials that are derived from animal or human sources. There are concerns about disease transmission, immunogenicity, and the ethics of sourcing these materials, which must be carefully navigated.

Lastly, the sustainability of biomaterials is becoming increasingly important. There is a growing need for materials that are not only effective and safe but also environmentally friendly and sustainable in the long term. This includes considering the entire lifecycle of the material, from production to disposal.

In conclusion, while biomaterials hold immense potential for advancing medical treatments, the challenges in developing them are substantial and multifaceted. Addressing these challenges requires a multidisciplinary approach, combining expertise from biology, chemistry, materials science, engineering, and ethics to create the next generation of biomaterials that are safe, effective, and sustainable.

Improving biocompatibility testing is crucial for the development of medical devices and materials that are safe and effective for human use. Researchers can enhance these testing methods by incorporating a multidisciplinary approach that leverages advancements in technology, materials science, and biology. One key area is the use of computational modeling and simulations to predict how materials will interact with biological systems, which can reduce the reliance on animal testing and streamline the development process.

The integration of high-throughput screening methods can also expedite the evaluation of biomaterials by allowing simultaneous testing of multiple material compositions and surface modifications. This can quickly generate large datasets that provide insights into the biocompatibility profiles of various materials. Additionally, adopting more sophisticated in vitro models that closely mimic human physiology, such as organ-on-a-chip systems, can provide a more accurate assessment of a material's performance in the body.

Chemical characterization is another critical aspect of biocompatibility testing. Improvements in analytical techniques, such as mass spectrometry and nuclear magnetic resonance spectroscopy, can offer more detailed information about the composition and potential leachable of biomaterials. This information is essential for assessing the safety of materials intended for medical use.

Furthermore, researchers can focus on developing standardized protocols for biocompatibility testing, which would facilitate comparison of results across different studies and improve the reproducibility of tests. This standardization can be achieved through collaboration with regulatory bodies and international standards organizations.

The use of bioinformatics and data analytics can also play a significant role in improving biocompatibility testing. By analyzing patterns and correlations within large datasets, researchers can identify potential biomarkers of compatibility or toxicity, leading to more targeted and efficient testing strategies.

Another approach is to enhance the sensitivity of biocompatibility tests by using more refined detection methods that can identify even low levels of adverse reactions. This could involve the development of new assays that can detect subtle changes in cell behavior or molecular markers indicative of an immune response.

Ethical considerations are also paramount in biocompatibility testing. Researchers must ensure that their testing methods are not only effective but also ethical, minimizing the use of animal testing where possible and adhering to the principles of the 3Rs (Replacement, Reduction, and Refinement).

In addition, researchers can improve biocompatibility testing by fostering closer collaboration between academia, industry, and regulatory agencies. This collaboration can lead to a more comprehensive understanding of the requirements for biocompatibility and the development of more predictive testing models.

Lastly, ongoing education and training for researchers in the latest biocompatibility testing methods and regulations are essential. This ensures that the scientific community remains up to date with the most current and effective practices, ultimately leading to safer and more reliable biomaterials for medical applications.

In summary, improving biocompatibility testing involves a combination of advanced scientific techniques, standardization of protocols, ethical considerations, and collaborative efforts across various sectors. By addressing these areas, researchers can significantly enhance the safety and efficacy of biomaterials used in medicine, leading to better patient outcomes and the advancement of healthcare technologies.

Computational modeling for biocompatibility presents several challenges that researchers must navigate to effectively predict material interactions with biological systems. One of the primary challenges is the complexity of biological systems, which are highly variable and subject to a multitude of factors that can influence outcomes. This complexity makes it difficult to create models that can accurately simulate the nuanced interactions between biomaterials and living tissues.

Another significant challenge is the need for extensive data to inform the models. Computational models require detailed information about the chemical and physical properties of materials, as well as data on how these materials interact with biological systems. However, such data is often scarce or incomplete, which can limit the accuracy of the models.

The scale of biological processes also poses a challenge. Biological interactions occur at various scales, from the molecular to the organ level, and computational models must be able to account for phenomena at each of these levels. This multiscale modeling is complex and computationally intensive, requiring sophisticated algorithms and significant computational power.

Moreover, the dynamic nature of biological systems means that models must be able to simulate changes over time, such as the degradation of materials or the healing process of tissues. Capturing these temporal dynamics is essential for predicting long-term biocompatibility but adds another layer of complexity to the modeling process.

Inter-individual variability is another hurdle. Each person's biological response to a material can be different, influenced by factors such as genetics, health status, and environmental exposures. Computational models must therefore be able to account for this variability to be broadly applicable, which is a challenging task given the current understanding of these factors.

Ethical considerations also come into play when using computational models for biocompatibility. While these models can reduce the need for animal testing, they cannot yet fully replace it. Ensuring that the models are ethically developed and used is an ongoing concern for the research community.

The integration of computational models with experimental data is also challenging. Models need to be validated and refined based on experimental results, which requires a seamless integration of computational and laboratory work. This interdisciplinary approach is essential but can be difficult to achieve due to differences in methodologies and expertise.

Furthermore, the regulatory acceptance of computational models is still evolving. Regulatory agencies require robust evidence to support the safety and efficacy of new materials, and computational models are just one part of this evidence. Gaining regulatory acceptance for models as a substitute for traditional biocompatibility testing is a complex process that involves demonstrating the reliability and validity of the models.

Lastly, the development of computational models for biocompatibility is a rapidly advancing field, and keeping up with the latest advancements in modeling techniques and computational technologies is a challenge. Researchers must continuously update their skills and knowledge to stay at the forefront of the field.

In summary, while computational modeling holds great promise for advancing the field of biocompatibility, it is not without its challenges. Addressing these challenges requires a concerted effort from researchers, clinicians, regulatory bodies, and the broader scientific community to develop reliable, accurate, and ethically sound models that can improve the safety and effectiveness of biomaterials in medicine.

Recent breakthroughs in computational modeling for biocompatibility have significantly advanced the field, offering new insights and tools for the development of medical devices and materials. One notable advancement is the use of computer simulations to replace in-vivo experiments for implantable medical devices. This shift towards in-silico research allows for a more ethical approach to testing and can accelerate the innovation process while reducing costs.

In the realm of cerebral circulation, computational models have been refined to simulate blood flow rate and regulatory mechanisms with greater accuracy. These models are now being used as pre-clinical tools, providing valuable predictions about how implantable devices will perform within the human body.

Another significant development is the integration of different methodologies in the study of biomolecular complexes. Researchers have employed coarse-grained (CG) modeling techniques, such as the GōMartini approach, to explore the nano mechanics of protein complexes. This has led to the first-ever CG modeling of an entire cell, which is a monumental step in understanding cellular behavior and interactions.

The AdResS method, which couples different molecular resolutions, has also been a breakthrough in computational modeling. It allows for the study of double-stranded DNA and other complex molecular systems, providing a more comprehensive view of biomolecular interactions.

Machine learning has been increasingly incorporated into computational modeling, enhancing the ability to predict biocompatibility by analyzing patterns in large datasets. This approach has improved the precision of biocompatibility assessments and has the potential to tailor medical devices to individual patient needs.

In addition to these modeling advancements, there have been strides in the development of in vitro analytical technologies. These technologies are used to characterize the biocompatibility of bioinks in 3D environments, which is crucial for the success of 3D bioprinting applications in tissue engineering.

The review of coronary stent biomechanics and biomaterials has also highlighted the value of computational modeling. Investigations into stent deployment, fracture, and drug-release mechanisms have provided deeper insights into stent performance. This knowledge is essential for improving stent technology and optimizing their design for better patient outcomes.

These breakthroughs in computational modeling are not just academic exercises; they have practical implications for the healthcare industry. By improving the predictability and reliability of biocompatibility assessments, computational modeling is helping to bring safer, more effective medical devices to the market more quickly. This progress is crucial for advancing patient care and represents a significant step forward in the intersection of technology and medicine.

The integration of machine learning into biocompatibility modeling can be further enhanced by focusing on several key areas. Firstly, the development of more sophisticated algorithms that can handle the complexity of biological systems is essential. These algorithms must be capable of processing and analyzing the vast amounts of data generated by biocompatibility studies, including genomic, proteomic, and metabolomic data. Machine learning can be used to identify patterns and relationships within this data that may not be apparent through traditional analysis methods.

Secondly, the creation of comprehensive databases that compile biocompatibility-related data from various sources would provide a valuable resource for machine learning models. These databases should include information on material properties, biological responses, and clinical outcomes. By training machine learning models on this diverse dataset, researchers can improve the predictive accuracy of biocompatibility assessments.

Another area of focus is the improvement of data quality and standardization. Machine learning models are only as good as the data they are trained on, so ensuring that the data is of high quality and standardized across studies is crucial. This may involve developing new protocols for data collection and processing, as well as guidelines for reporting biocompatibility results.

The use of machine learning in the design of experiments can also be expanded. By analyzing previous experimental results, machine learning models can suggest optimal conditions for new biocompatibility tests, potentially reducing the number of experiments needed and accelerating the research process.

Furthermore, machine learning can be integrated into the regulatory approval process for new biomaterials. By demonstrating that machine learning models can reliably predict biocompatibility, these models could be used to supplement or even replace certain aspects of the regulatory testing requirements, streamlining the approval process.

Collaboration between computational scientists, biologists, and materials scientists is vital for the successful integration of machine learning into biocompatibility modeling. Interdisciplinary teams can work together to ensure that machine learning models are informed by the latest scientific knowledge and that they accurately reflect the complexities of biological systems.

The ethical implications of using machine learning in biocompatibility modeling must also be considered. As machine learning models play a larger role in the development of medical devices and materials, it is important to ensure that these models are transparent and that their predictions can be explained and justified.

Lastly, the ongoing education and training of researchers in the latest machine learning techniques will ensure that the potential of these tools is fully realized in the field of biocompatibility modeling. By staying abreast of the latest developments in machine learning, researchers can continue to refine and improve their models, leading to more accurate and reliable predictions of biocompatibility.

In the field of biocompatibility modeling, machine learning algorithms play a pivotal role in analyzing and predicting how materials interact with biological systems. Specific algorithms that have been employed include AdaBoost, which is a boosting algorithm that combines multiple weak learners to create a strong classifier. This algorithm is particularly useful for classification tasks where it's important to minimize errors. Artificial Neural Networks (ANNs) are also widely used; these are inspired by the biological neural networks and can capture complex patterns in data through their interconnected layers of nodes. ANNs are especially beneficial in modeling non-linear relationships, which are common in biological systems.

Another algorithm is the Naïve Bayes classifier, which applies Bayes' theorem with the assumption of independence between the features. It's known for its simplicity and effectiveness, particularly in large datasets. Decision Trees are another method, which model decisions and their possible consequences as a tree-like structure, making them intuitive and easy to interpret. Support Vector Machines (SVMs) are also utilized for their ability to find the optimal boundary between different classes, which is crucial in determining biocompatibility.

K-Nearest Neighbors (KNN) is a non-parametric algorithm that classifies data based on the majority vote of its neighbors, with the object being assigned to the class most common among its k nearest neighbors. This method is particularly useful when there is little or no prior knowledge about the distribution of the data.

Furthermore, machine learning models like Random Forests, which are an ensemble of decision trees, are used to improve predictive accuracy and control over-fitting. Gradient Boosting Machines (GBMs) are another ensemble technique that builds models in a stage-wise fashion and are used for both regression and classification problems.

Deep Learning, a subset of machine learning, has also made significant contributions to biocompatibility modeling. Convolutional Neural Networks (CNNs), a class of deep neural networks, are particularly effective in analyzing visual imagery and are used in biocompatibility studies involving imaging data. Recurrent Neural Networks (RNNs), known for their ability to process sequences of data, are useful in modeling time-dependent or sequential data, such as changes in tissue response over time.

Moreover, the integration of machine learning with other computational methods, such as molecular dynamics simulations, has led to more accurate and comprehensive models. For instance, the combination of machine learning with quantum mechanics/molecular mechanics (QM/MM) approaches has provided insights into the molecular-level interactions between biomaterials and biological environments.

The use of machine learning in biocompatibility modeling is not limited to these algorithms. Researchers continuously explore and develop new methods to improve the predictive power and efficiency of these models. As the field advances, we can expect to see the adoption of more sophisticated algorithms that can handle the increasing complexity and volume of data in biocompatibility studies.

Addressing the interpretability and transparency of machine learning models for regulatory purposes is a multifaceted challenge that requires a concerted effort from various stakeholders, including data scientists, regulatory bodies, and industry practitioners. The goal is to ensure that machine learning models are not just effective but also understandable and trustworthy. One approach is to implement model-agnostic interpretation techniques that provide insights into model behavior without relying on the internal workings of the models themselves. Techniques such as partial dependence plots (PDPs), individual conditional expectation (ICE) plots, and accumulated local effects (ALE) plots can help visualize the relationship between features and the model's predictions.

Another strategy is to use inherently interpretable models whenever possible. Models like linear regression, decision trees, and rule-based systems may offer less complexity but are easier to understand and explain. For more complex models, such as deep neural networks, developing methods to approximate their predictions with simpler, interpretable models can be beneficial. This can involve techniques like Local Interpretable Model-agnostic Explanations (LIME) or SHapley Additive exPlanations (SHAP), which explain individual predictions by approximating the local decision boundary.

Transparency can also be enhanced by documenting the entire machine learning pipeline, from data collection and preprocessing to model training and validation. This documentation should include details about the datasets used, feature selection processes, model parameters, and performance metrics. Such comprehensive documentation can help regulatory bodies assess the reliability and fairness of the models.

Moreover, engaging domain experts in the model development process can improve interpretability. Experts can provide valuable insights into which features are most relevant and how they should influence the model's decisions. This domain knowledge can be incorporated into the model either directly, through feature engineering, or indirectly, by guiding the model selection and tuning process.

The development of standards and guidelines for interpretability and transparency is also crucial. Regulatory bodies can work with industry and academic leaders to establish clear criteria for what constitutes an interpretable and transparent model in different contexts. These standards can then be used to evaluate and certify models before they are deployed in sensitive applications.

Furthermore, fostering a culture of ethical AI development is essential. This involves prioritizing interpretability and transparency from the outset of a project, rather than treating them as afterthoughts. Ethical considerations should be integrated into the design and implementation of machine learning models, ensuring that they align with societal values and legal requirements.

The use of post-hoc interpretation methods can also be helpful, especially for complex models that cannot be interpretable by design. Post-hoc techniques can provide explanations after the model has made a prediction, helping to shed light on the reasoning behind specific decisions. However, these methods should be used with caution, as they can sometimes lead to misleading or incorrect interpretations.

Another important aspect is the communication of model interpretations. Data scientists must be able to explain their models to non-technical stakeholders, including regulators, in a clear and accessible manner. This may involve creating visualizations, summaries, or interactive tools that allow users to explore the model's behavior.

Finally, ongoing research and development in the field of explainable AI (XAI) are vital. As machine learning models become more complex, new methods for interpretation and transparency will need to be developed. Collaborative research efforts between academia and industry can accelerate the discovery of innovative solutions that meet the evolving needs of regulatory bodies and society at large.

In conclusion, addressing the interpretability and transparency of machine learning models for regulatory purposes is a complex task that requires a multi-pronged approach. It involves the use of interpretation techniques, engagement with domain experts, comprehensive documentation, development of standards, ethical AI development, post-hoc methods, effective communication, and ongoing research. By tackling these challenges, we can build machine learning systems that are not only powerful but also responsible and trustworthy.

Ensuring that interpretability methods do not compromise the performance of machine learning models is a critical aspect of model development, particularly in regulated environments where both accuracy and transparency are required. One approach is to select inherently interpretable models that provide a good balance between performance and understandability, such as linear regression or decision trees, which are straightforward to interpret and can often achieve high performance in many tasks. When using more complex models, techniques like LIME (Local Interpretable Model-agnostic Explanations) or SHAP (SHapley Additive exPlanations) can be applied to interpret model predictions without altering the model itself, thus maintaining the original performance.

Another strategy is to incorporate interpretability as a criterion during the model selection and training process. This can involve using regularization techniques that not only prevent overfitting but also promote simpler models that are easier to interpret. Additionally, feature engineering can play a significant role in interpretability; by carefully selecting and transforming features, data scientists can improve both the model's performance and the ease with which its decisions can be understood.

The development of hybrid models that combine the strengths of both interpretable and complex models is also a promising approach. These models can use a complex algorithm to achieve high accuracy while employing a simpler, interpretable model to approximate and explain the predictions of the complex model.

Moreover, the field of explainable artificial intelligence (XAI) is actively researching new methods and algorithms that aim to improve the interpretability of machine learning models without sacrificing performance. This includes the development of new types of neural networks that are designed to be more transparent, such as attention mechanisms or networks with built-in explanation capabilities.

It is also important to evaluate the interpretability methods themselves to ensure they do not introduce biases or inaccuracies. This can be done through rigorous testing and validation on independent datasets, as well as by seeking feedback from domain experts who can assess the plausibility and relevance of the explanations provided.

Furthermore, the use of post-hoc interpretation methods, which are applied after the model has been trained, can offer insights into the model's behavior without affecting its performance. These methods can help to identify the most important features and to understand the model's decision-making process on a case-by-case basis.

Transparency in the modeling process is crucial for regulatory acceptance. By maintaining detailed documentation of the model development process, including the rationale behind model choices and the methods used for interpretation, data scientists can provide the necessary evidence to demonstrate that the model is both accurate and interpretable.

Lastly, ongoing research and collaboration between academia, industry, and regulatory bodies can help to establish best practices and guidelines for developing models that meet both performance and interpretability standards. This collaborative effort can lead to the creation of benchmarks and frameworks that facilitate the development of models that are both high-performing and transparent.

In conclusion, ensuring that interpretability methods do not compromise model performance involves a combination of choosing the right models, applying appropriate interpretation techniques, incorporating interpretability into the model development process, evaluating and validating interpretation methods, maintaining transparency, and engaging in ongoing research and collaboration. By addressing these aspects, it is possible to develop machine learning models that are both effective and understandable, thereby meeting the needs of various stakeholders, including regulators, practitioners, and end-users.

The regulatory adoption of machine learning models has seen several successful examples, particularly in the financial sector. One of the most prominent areas is in anti-money laundering (AML) efforts, where machine learning models have been deployed to enhance the detection and reporting of suspicious activities. For instance, financial institutions have utilized machine learning strategies to analyze transaction data more effectively, identifying patterns that may indicate money laundering with greater accuracy and efficiency than traditional rule-based systems.

In the realm of regulatory compliance, machine learning models have been instrumental in improving the efficiency and effectiveness of Know Your Customer (KYC) processes. By automating the analysis of customer data, these models have significantly reduced the time and resources required for KYC checks, while also minimizing the risk of human error.

Another area where machine learning has been successfully integrated is in fraud detection. Banks and financial institutions are leveraging advanced algorithms to monitor transactions in real-time, flagging potential fraud more quickly and accurately. This proactive approach has not only helped in preventing financial losses but also in maintaining customer trust and regulatory compliance.

Machine learning models have also been adopted for market surveillance, where they are used to detect and prevent market manipulation and insider trading. By analyzing vast amounts of trading data, these models can identify suspicious patterns and alert regulatory authorities, contributing to fairer and more transparent financial markets.

Moreover, in the healthcare sector, machine learning models have been used to predict patient outcomes, personalize treatment plans, and manage healthcare resources more efficiently. Regulatory bodies have recognized the potential of these models to improve patient care and have begun to incorporate them into the approval processes for new drugs and medical devices.

These examples demonstrate the growing trust in machine learning models by regulatory bodies and their potential to transform various industries by enhancing compliance, efficiency, and decision-making processes. As machine learning technology continues to evolve, it is likely that its regulatory adoption will expand into even more sectors, further revolutionizing the way organizations operate and comply with regulations.

Ensuring the fairness and accountability of machine learning models in regulatory contexts is a multifaceted challenge that requires a comprehensive approach. Fairness in machine learning involves creating algorithms that make decisions without biases that disadvantage any group or individual. To achieve this, it's essential to have diverse datasets that are representative of all groups affected by the model's decisions. This helps to prevent biases that could be present in training data from perpetuating or amplifying existing inequalities. Moreover, fairness must be defined and measured according to the context in which the model operates, considering the various dimensions of fairness and the trade-offs between them.

Accountability in machine learning refers to the ability to trace and justify the decisions made by algorithms. This involves creating transparent systems where the decision-making process can be understood and scrutinized by regulators and stakeholders. Machine learning models should be designed with explainability in mind, allowing for clear communication of how decisions are made. This is particularly important in regulatory contexts where decisions can have significant impacts on individuals and communities.

One approach to ensuring fairness and accountability is through the development and enforcement of regulatory standards. These standards can provide guidelines for the ethical development and deployment of machine learning models, including requirements for transparency, data quality, and algorithmic auditing. Collaborative efforts between lawmakers, industry experts, and academia can lead to the creation of such standards, which can be tailored to specific sectors and applications.

Algorithmic auditing is another crucial component. Independent reviews of machine learning models can assess their fairness and identify potential biases. Audits can also evaluate the models' compliance with regulatory standards and ethical principles. This process can be supported by tools and frameworks that facilitate the assessment of machine learning models, such as impact assessments and fairness metrics.

The use of interpretable machine learning models can also aid in ensuring fairness and accountability. Interpretable models allow for easier examination of the factors influencing decisions, making it simpler to identify and correct biases. When complex models are necessary, techniques like feature importance analysis and model-agnostic explanation methods can help to shed light on the model's behavior.

Continuous monitoring and updating of machine learning models are also essential. As data and societal norms evolve, models must be re-evaluated to ensure they continue to operate fairly and accountably. This includes reassessing the model's performance on new data, updating the model to reflect changes in the underlying population, and revising the model's objectives to align with current ethical standards.

Stakeholder engagement is another key aspect. Involving the individuals and communities affected by machine learning decisions in the development and oversight process can provide valuable perspectives on what constitutes fairness and how accountability should be maintained. This participatory approach can help to build trust and ensure that the models serve the interests of all stakeholders.

Education and training for those involved in the development and deployment of machine learning models are also critical. This includes not only data scientists and engineers but also regulators and policymakers who need to understand the capabilities and limitations of these technologies. A well-informed workforce can better navigate the ethical and regulatory challenges associated with machine learning.

Lastly, international collaboration can play a role in harmonizing standards and practices across borders. As machine learning models are often deployed globally, international cooperation can help to ensure that fairness and accountability are maintained consistently, regardless of where the model is used.

In conclusion, ensuring the fairness and accountability of machine learning models in regulatory contexts is a complex endeavor that requires careful consideration of ethical principles, rigorous technical approaches, and ongoing collaboration among various stakeholders. By addressing these challenges holistically, we can harness the benefits of machine learning while safeguarding against potential harms.

Addressing the interpretability and transparency of machine learning models for regulatory purposes is a critical concern that intersects with the fields of artificial intelligence (AI), law, and ethics. Interpretability refers to the extent to which a human can understand the cause of a decision made by a machine learning model, while transparency involves the openness of the AI system in terms of its design, operation, and data processing. To ensure that machine learning models are both interpretable and transparent, several strategies can be employed.

Firstly, it is essential to adopt model-agnostic interpretation techniques. These techniques, such as partial dependence plots (PDPs), individual conditional expectation (ICE) plots, and accumulated local effects (ALE) plots, provide insights into the model's behavior without depending on its internal mechanisms. They can help visualize how changes in input features affect the model's predictions, thereby offering a window into the model's decision-making process.

Secondly, the use of inherently interpretable models, whenever possible, is advisable. Models like linear regression, decision trees, and rule-based systems may offer less complexity but are easier to understand and explain. For more complex models, such as deep neural networks, developing methods to approximate their predictions with simpler, interpretable models can be beneficial. Techniques like Local Interpretable Model-agnostic Explanations (LIME) or SHapley Additive exPlanations (SHAP) can explain individual predictions by approximating the local decision boundary.

Thirdly, comprehensive documentation of the machine learning pipeline is crucial. This includes details about the datasets used, feature selection processes, model parameters, and performance metrics. Such documentation can help regulatory bodies assess the reliability and fairness of the models.

Fourthly, engaging domain experts in the model development process can improve interpretability. Experts can provide valuable insights into which features are most relevant and how they should influence the model's decisions. This domain knowledge can be incorporated into the model either directly, through feature engineering, or indirectly, by guiding the model selection and tuning process.

Fifthly, the development of standards and guidelines for interpretability and transparency is also crucial. Regulatory bodies can work with industry and academic leaders to establish clear criteria for what constitutes an interpretable and transparent model in different contexts. These standards can then be used to evaluate and certify models before they are deployed in sensitive applications.

Sixthly, algorithmic auditing is another critical component. Independent reviews of machine learning models can assess their fairness and identify potential biases. Audits can also evaluate the models' compliance with regulatory standards and ethical principles.

Seventhly, continuous monitoring and updating of machine learning models are also essential. As data and societal norms evolve, models must be re-evaluated to ensure they continue to operate fairly and accountably.

Eighthly, stakeholder engagement is another key aspect. Involving the individuals and communities affected by machine learning decisions in the development and oversight process can provide valuable perspectives on what constitutes fairness and how accountability should be maintained.

Ninthly, education and training for those involved in the development and deployment of machine learning models are also critical. This includes not only data scientists and engineers but also regulators and policymakers who need to understand the capabilities and limitations of these technologies.

Lastly, international collaboration can play a role in harmonizing standards and practices across borders. As machine learning models are often deployed globally, international cooperation can help to ensure that fairness and accountability are maintained consistently, regardless of where the model is used.

In conclusion, addressing the interpretability and transparency of machine learning models for regulatory purposes is a complex task that requires a multi-pronged approach. It involves the use of interpretation techniques, engagement with domain experts, comprehensive documentation, development of standards, ethical AI development, post-hoc methods, effective communication, and ongoing research. By tackling these challenges, we can build machine learning systems that are not only powerful but also responsible and trustworthy.

Progress in Treating the Undruggable:

From cancer to neurodegenerative diseases, scientists are making strides in targeting previously challenging conditions. Novel approaches, such as protein degradation techniques and precision medicine, offer hope for patients.

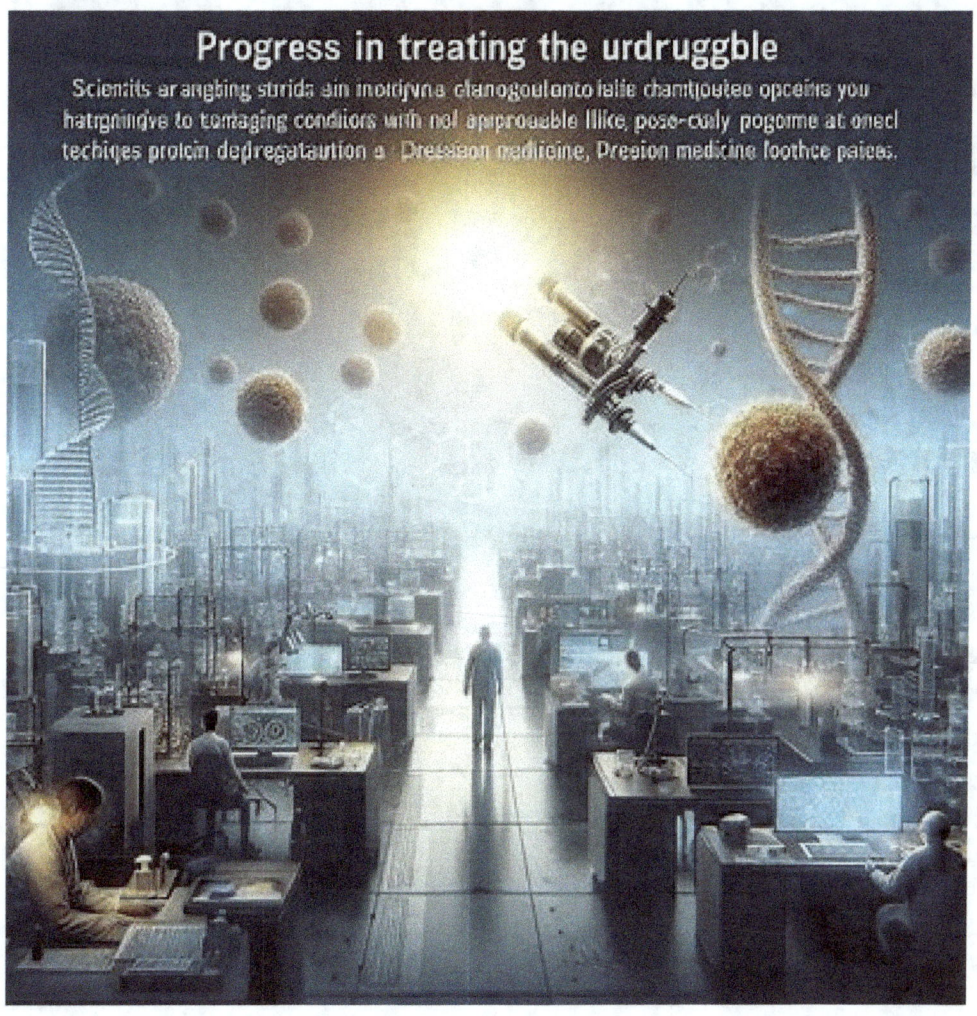

The concept of 'undruggable' targets has long presented a formidable challenge in the treatment of complex diseases, particularly in the realm of oncology. These targets are typically crucial proteins or biomolecules that are integral to disease progression but have eluded intervention with existing therapies. The term 'undruggable' often refers to proteins with essential roles in signaling pathways, structural functions, or gene regulation that lack well-defined binding sites for traditional small molecule drugs. However, recent advancements in biomedical research and drug discovery are beginning to shift this paradigm.

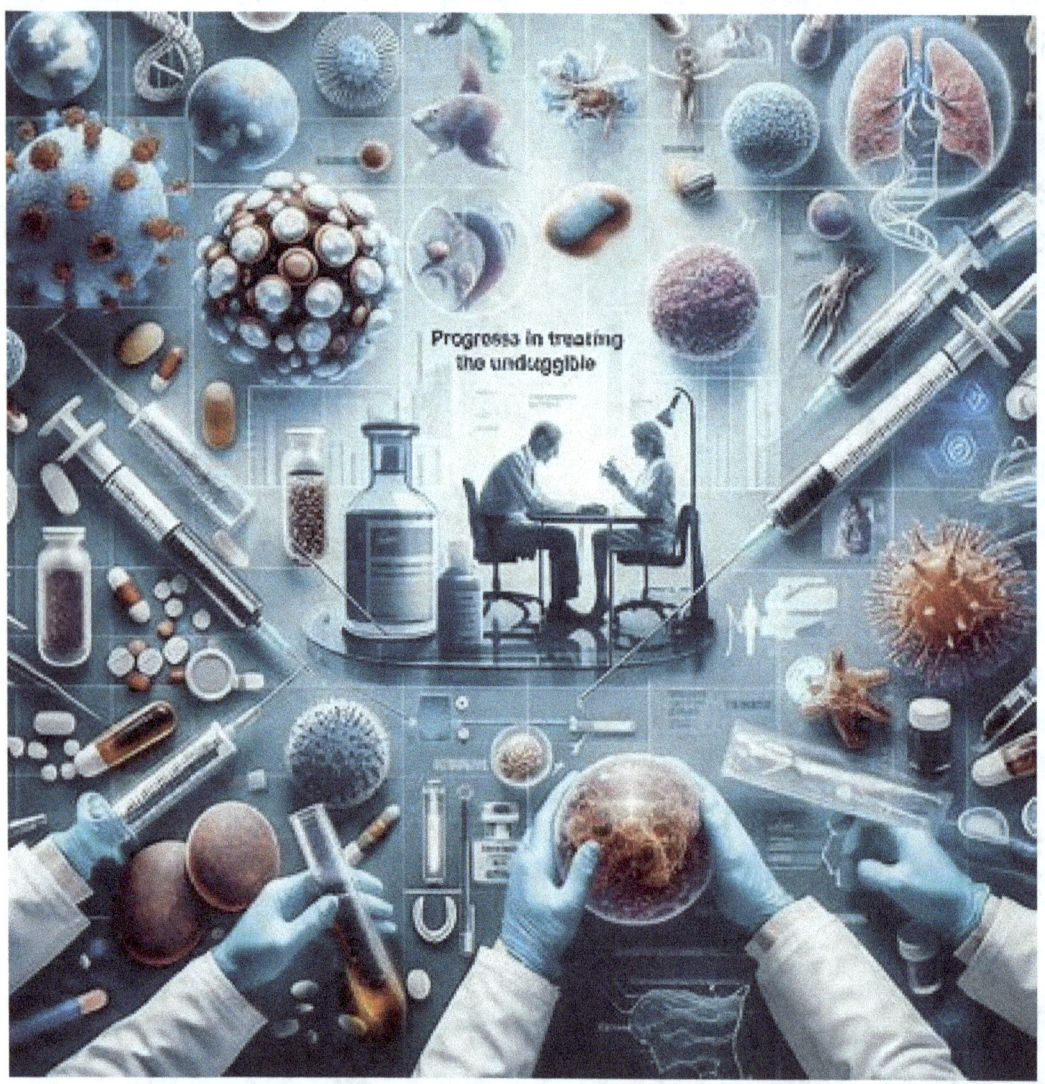

Innovative strategies such as targeted protein degradation (TPD) have emerged, harnessing the cell's own machinery to selectively eliminate disease-causing proteins. This approach has shown promise in addressing proteins that were previously considered undruggable due to their structure or the nature of their interaction with other proteins. TPD leverages small molecules known as

PROTACs (proteolysis-targeting chimeras) or molecular glues to tag these problematic proteins for degradation by the ubiquitin-proteasome system.

Precision medicine is another frontier pushing the boundaries of what is considered treatable. By tailoring treatment to the individual genetic makeup of a patient's disease, precision medicine can identify unique vulnerabilities in cancer cells that may be exploited for therapeutic intervention. This personalized approach often involves comprehensive genomic profiling to uncover specific mutations or alterations that drive disease progression, enabling the development of targeted therapies that can more effectively combat these conditions.

Moreover, the field of drug discovery has seen a surge in the use of chemically induced proximity, a technique that facilitates the interaction between molecules that would otherwise not come into contact. This method has been instrumental in the development of drugs targeting the RAS family of proteins, notorious for their role in cancer and their previous classification as undruggable.

The advent of CRISPR technology and whole-genome screening has also accelerated the identification of new therapeutic targets. These advanced techniques allow for the functional characterization of genes and the elucidation of their roles in disease, providing a broader landscape of potential targets for drug development.

Furthermore, the concept of druggability is evolving with the advancement of technology. What was once deemed undruggable may now be within reach thanks to the development of novel drug modalities and the redefinition of draggability based on current technological capabilities. As such, the term 'difficult to drug' or 'yet to be drugged' may be more appropriate, reflecting the progress and potential for future breakthroughs in treating these challenging targets.

The fight against neurodegenerative diseases has also benefited from these advances. For instance, targeting the mRNA of proteins involved in conditions like Parkinson's disease has opened new avenues for intervention. Small molecule binders and degraders that can interact with mRNA offer a groundbreaking approach to modulating the expression of proteins that were previously inaccessible.

In summary, the landscape of drug discovery and treatment is undergoing a significant transformation. The concerted efforts of scientists and the integration of emerging technologies are making it possible to target the undruggable, offering renewed hope for patients suffering from a range of debilitating conditions. As research continues to advance, it is likely that the list of undruggable targets will shrink, heralding a new era of therapeutic possibilities.

Targeted protein degradation (TPD) is a revolutionary approach in drug discovery that aims to eliminate disease-causing proteins from within cells. Unlike traditional drugs that inhibit protein function, TPD strategies seek to remove problematic proteins altogether. This is achieved by harnessing the cell's natural degradation pathways, such as the ubiquitin-proteasome system (UPS) and lysosomal pathways.

The ubiquitin-proteasome system plays a critical role in maintaining cellular protein homeostasis by degrading misfolded, damaged, or unneeded proteins. In this system, proteins are tagged with ubiquitin, a small regulatory protein, which signals for their degradation by the proteasome, a large protein complex responsible for protein breakdown. TPD technologies, such as Proteolysis Targeting Chimeras (PROTACs), utilize this system by bringing together the target protein with an E3 ubiquitin ligase, facilitating the transfer of ubiquitin and subsequent degradation of the target protein.

PROTACs are bifunctional molecules composed of two binding domains connected by a linker: one domain binds to the target protein, and the other to an E3 ligase. This proximity induces the transfer of ubiquitin from the ligase to the target protein, marking it for degradation. PROTACs are highly selective, offering the advantage of targeting specific proteins while sparing others, which can reduce off-target effects and improve therapeutic outcomes.

Another TPD strategy involves molecular glues, small molecules that promote the interaction between the target protein and an E3 ligase, leading to ubiquitination and degradation. Unlike PROTACs, molecular glues do not require a direct binding domain for the target protein, which can be beneficial for targeting proteins without well-defined binding pockets.

Lysosome-Targeting Chimeras (LYTACs) represent a different approach, directing proteins to the lysosome, an organelle responsible for degrading long-lived proteins and larger cellular components. LYTACs can target extracellular and membrane proteins, expanding the scope of TPD beyond the intracellular proteins addressed by PROTACs and molecular glues.

The development of TPD has been bolstered by advancements in understanding the structural biology of proteins and the mechanisms of protein-protein interactions. High-throughput screening methods and computational modeling have also played a role in identifying potential TPD candidates.

Clinical trials are currently underway for several TPD compounds, with a focus on oncology, where the need to target traditionally undruggable proteins is particularly acute. The success of these trials could lead to a new generation of cancer therapies that offer more effective and less toxic treatment options.

In addition to cancer, TPD has potential applications in other diseases characterized by aberrant protein function or accumulation, such as neurodegenerative disorders. By removing proteins that contribute to disease pathology, TPD offers a novel therapeutic strategy that could complement or replace traditional small molecule inhibitors.

The field of TPD is rapidly evolving, with ongoing research into new ligases, degradation pathways, and target proteins. As our understanding of the underlying biology expands, so too does the potential for TPD to transform the treatment of a wide range of diseases.

In conclusion, targeted protein degradation represents a significant shift in the paradigm of drug development. By leveraging the cell's own mechanisms for protein regulation, TPD provides a powerful tool for addressing some of the most challenging targets in medicine. With continued research and development, TPD may offer hope for patients with conditions that have long been considered untreatable.

The field of targeted protein degradation has seen significant advancements with the development of PROTACs, and several of these innovative molecules have progressed into clinical trials. For instance, ARV-110 and ARV-471 are two PROTACs that have shown excellent efficacy in phase II clinical trials. ARV-110 is designed to target the androgen receptor (AR), which plays a pivotal role in the progression of prostate cancer. By promoting the degradation of the AR protein, ARV-110 aims to halt the growth of cancer cells that depend on this receptor for survival.

Similarly, ARV-471 is a PROTAC that targets the estrogen receptor (ER), which is crucial in the development and progression of certain types of breast cancer. By degrading the ER protein, ARV-471 seeks to impede the proliferation of cancer cells that require this receptor. These two examples represent a promising step forward in the application of PROTAC technology in oncology, offering potential new therapies for patients with hormone receptor-positive cancers.

Other examples of PROTACs that have reached clinical trials include those targeting Bruton's tyrosine kinase (BTK), Bromodomain-containing protein 4 (BRD4), Signal Transducer and Activator of Transcription 3 (STAT3), Interleukin-1 Receptor-Associated Kinase 4 (IRAK4), and the Tau protein. BTK is an essential enzyme in the B-cell receptor signaling pathway, and its degradation by PROTACs could provide a novel approach to treating B-cell malignancies. BRD4 is involved in regulating gene expression, and its targeting by PROTACs could have implications for various cancers and inflammatory diseases.

STAT3 is a transcription factor that, when dysregulated, can contribute to the development of cancer and immune disorders. PROTACs that degrade STAT3 could therefore offer a new strategy for treating these conditions. IRAK4 is a kinase involved in the innate immune response, and its degradation by PROTACs could be beneficial in treating inflammatory diseases and certain cancers. Lastly, the Tau protein is associated with neurodegenerative diseases like Alzheimer's, and PROTACs targeting Tau could potentially slow or halt the progression of these disorders.

These clinical trials are critical for determining the safety, efficacy, and optimal dosing of PROTACs in humans. The success of these trials will not only validate the therapeutic potential of PROTACs but also pave the way for the development of additional compounds targeting a broader range of proteins. As research continues, it is likely that more PROTACs will enter clinical trials, expanding the possibilities for treating diseases that have been challenging to address with traditional small molecule drugs.

PROTACs, or Proteolysis-Targeting Chimeras, are a class of therapeutic agents that operate on a unique principle of targeted protein degradation. Unlike traditional inhibitors that block the activity of proteins, PROTACs aim to completely remove specific proteins from the cell. This is achieved through the recruitment of the cell's ubiquitin-proteasome system (UPS), a natural cellular process responsible for protein degradation and turnover.

The mechanism of action for PROTACs involves three key components: the target protein, an E3 ubiquitin ligase, and the PROTAC molecule itself, which serves as a bridge between the target protein and the E3 ligase. The PROTAC molecule is bifunctional, with one end binding to the target protein and the other end to the E3 ligase. When the PROTAC molecule binds to the target protein, it also recruits the E3 ligase to form a ternary complex. This proximity allows the E3 ligase to transfer multiple ubiquitin molecules to the target protein.

Ubiquitination is a signal for the proteasome, a large protein complex, to recognize and degrade the tagged protein. The proteasome shreds the protein into small peptides, effectively removing the protein's function from the cell. What makes PROTACs particularly appealing is their catalytic mode of action; a single PROTAC molecule can induce the degradation of multiple target protein molecules, making them highly efficient.

Another advantage of PROTACs is their selectivity. Because they can be designed to bind to unique sites on target proteins, they can degrade specific proteins while leaving others untouched. This reduces the likelihood of off-target effects, which are a common problem with traditional small molecule drugs.

The versatility of PROTACs is also noteworthy. They can potentially target a wide range of proteins, including those that do not have enzymatic activity or are not located on the cell surface, which are typically considered 'undruggable' by conventional drugs. This opens new avenues for the treatment of diseases that have been difficult to address with existing therapies.

The development of PROTACs has been facilitated by advances in several scientific fields, including molecular biology, chemistry, and structural biology. Understanding the three-dimensional structure of proteins and the dynamics of protein-protein interactions has been crucial in designing effective PROTAC molecules.

Despite their potential, PROTACs also face challenges. One of the main hurdles is ensuring that they can enter cells and reach their target proteins, which often requires careful design to balance size, solubility, and permeability. Additionally, the development of resistance to PROTACs, as with any drug, is a concern that researchers are actively investigating.

In conclusion, PROTACs represent a transformative approach to drug design and therapy. By co-opting the cell's own degradation machinery, they offer a powerful means to eliminate disease-causing proteins with high specificity and efficiency. As research progresses, PROTACs may become a staple in the treatment of a variety of diseases, particularly those where conventional therapies have fallen short.

The design and optimization of PROTACs, or Proteolysis-Targeting Chimeras, are intricate processes that involve a deep understanding of molecular biology, chemistry, and pharmacology. The primary goal in designing a PROTAC is to create a molecule that can selectively bind to both a target protein and an E3 ubiquitin ligase, facilitating the ubiquitination and subsequent degradation of the target protein by the proteasome.

The process begins with the identification of a suitable ligand that can bind to the target protein with high specificity and affinity. This ligand serves as the 'warhead' of the PROTAC molecule. The next step is to select an appropriate E3 ligase recruiter, which is a molecule known to bind to one of the many E3 ubiquitin ligases within the cell. The choice of E3 ligase is crucial, as it must be capable of ubiquitinating the target protein once it is brought into proximity by the PROTAC.

Once the warhead and the E3 ligase recruiter have been identified, they are connected via a linker. The linker is not merely a passive scaffold; its length, flexibility, and composition can significantly affect the ability of the PROTAC to form a stable ternary complex with the target protein and the E3 ligase. The linker must be optimized to ensure that it positions the ligase for efficient transfer of ubiquitin to the target protein.

After the initial PROTAC molecule is synthesized, it undergoes a series of optimizations. This iterative process involves modifying the warhead, the linker, and the E3 ligase recruiter to improve the PROTAC's potency, selectivity, solubility, and permeability. High-throughput screening, structure-activity relationship (SAR) studies, and computational modeling are often employed to refine the design of the PROTAC.

One of the challenges in PROTAC design is ensuring that the molecule is cell-permeable so that it can reach intracellular targets. This often requires balancing the molecular weight and polarity of the PROTAC to facilitate its entry into cells without compromising its degradation activity. Another challenge is minimizing off-target effects, which can be addressed by enhancing the selectivity of the warhead and the E3 ligase recruiter.

Recent advancements have led to the development of new-generation PROTACs, which include small-molecule PROTAC prodrugs, biomacromolecule-PROTAC conjugates, and nano-PROTACs. These novel formats aim to overcome some of the limitations of traditional PROTACs, such as poor pharmacokinetics and off-target toxicity. For instance, PROTAC prodrugs can be designed to be activated only within the target tissue, reducing systemic exposure and side effects.

The optimization of PROTACs also involves evaluating their pharmacodynamic and pharmacokinetic properties. This includes assessing their stability, distribution, metabolism, and excretion in biological systems. Such evaluations are critical for determining the dosing regimen and potential for drug-drug interactions.

In addition to empirical testing, computational strategies such as molecular docking and virtual screening are increasingly used in the design and optimization of PROTACs. These techniques can predict how different modifications to the PROTAC structure will affect its interaction with the target protein and the E3 ligase, thereby guiding the optimization process.

As the field of targeted protein degradation continues to evolve, the design and optimization of PROTACs remain dynamic and innovative areas of research. The ongoing development of new chemistries, delivery methods, and computational tools is expected to further enhance the efficacy and applicability of PROTACs in treating a wide range of diseases.

The delivery of PROTACs (Proteolysis-Targeting Chimeras) to specific tissues is a complex challenge that is pivotal to their success as therapeutic agents. One of the primary hurdles is achieving the selective targeting of tissues while avoiding off-target effects. PROTACs need to reach and penetrate the cells of the targeted tissue in sufficient concentrations to exert their therapeutic effects without affecting healthy tissues. This requires a delicate balance of properties such as molecular size, solubility, and stability in the bloodstream.

Another significant challenge is the optimization of the PROTACs' pharmacokinetic (PK) and pharmacodynamic (PD) profiles. These molecules must have a favorable distribution within the body, a suitable half-life to allow for appropriate dosing intervals, and the ability to be metabolized and excreted safely. The inherent physicochemical characteristics of PROTACs, which often include large molecular weights and complex structures due to their bifunctional nature, can impede their ability to diffuse through cell membranes and reach intracellular targets.

Furthermore, the serum stability of PROTACs is crucial for their effectiveness. If a PROTAC is rapidly degraded or inactivated in the bloodstream, it may not reach the target tissue in active form, or it may necessitate higher doses, increasing the risk of side effects. The development of delivery systems that can protect PROTACs from premature degradation while facilitating their release at the target site is an area of ongoing research.

The specificity of E3 ligases, which are integral to the mechanism of action of PROTACs, also poses a challenge. Currently, only a limited number of E3 ligases are utilized in PROTAC design, but the human body has over 600 E3 ligases, some of which are expressed in tissue-specific patterns. Exploiting these tissue-specific ligases could enhance the precision of PROTAC delivery, ensuring that the degradation of target proteins occurs only where needed.

Additionally, the development of resistance to PROTACs is a potential issue. Tumor heterogeneity and the ability of cancer cells to adapt and develop resistance mechanisms could reduce the long-term efficacy of PROTACs. Strategies to overcome resistance may include the design of PROTACs that can target multiple degradation pathways or the combination of PROTACs with other therapeutic agents.

The cellular uptake of PROTACs is another area that requires attention. While some cells may readily internalize these molecules, others may be less permeable, necessitating the development of strategies to enhance cellular uptake, such as the use of cell-penetrating peptides or other delivery vectors.

Lastly, the potential immunogenicity of PROTACs cannot be overlooked. As foreign substances, they may elicit an immune response, which could not only diminish their therapeutic effect but also pose safety concerns. Ensuring that PROTACs are designed to minimize immunogenicity is essential for their successful clinical application.

In conclusion, while PROTACs represent a promising new class of therapeutics with the potential to target previously 'undruggable' proteins, the challenges in their delivery to specific tissues are multifaceted and require innovative solutions. Addressing these challenges is critical for the translation of PROTAC technology from the laboratory to the clinic, where it has the potential to significantly impact the treatment of various diseases.

Exploiting tissue-specific ligases for PROTAC delivery is a sophisticated strategy that leverages the unique expression patterns of E3 ubiquitin ligases across different tissues. E3 ligases are enzymes that catalyze the transfer of ubiquitin to specific substrate proteins, marking them for degradation by the proteasome. Since different tissues may express distinct sets of E3 ligases, identifying ligases that are predominantly active in a target tissue can enhance the selectivity and reduce off-target effects of PROTACs.

The development of PROTACs that are selective for tissue-specific ligases involves comprehensive research to map the expression profiles of E3 ligases across various tissues. This information can guide the selection of an appropriate E3 ligase that is highly expressed in the disease-affected tissue but has low expression in healthy tissues. By designing PROTACs that recruit these tissue-specific ligases, researchers can direct the degradation of disease-causing proteins primarily in the target tissue.

Moreover, the tissue-specific nature of certain E3 ligases can be exploited to develop PROTACs that are activated only in the presence of the ligase. This approach ensures that the PROTAC remains inactive until it reaches the tissue where the ligase is present, thereby minimizing systemic exposure and potential side effects. For example, the E3 ligase MDM2 is abundant in certain tumor tissues, and PROTACs designed to target MDM2 can provide a more focused treatment for cancers expressing this ligase.

Another aspect of utilizing tissue-specific ligases is the design of PROTACs with linkers that are optimized for the spatial requirements of the ligase-protein interaction. The length and composition of the linker can influence the formation of the ternary complex between the PROTAC, the target protein, and the E3 ligase. Fine-tuning the linker can enhance the degradation of the target protein specifically in tissues where the chosen ligase is active.

The bifunctional nature of PROTACs also allows for the incorporation of ligand moieties that have inherent tissue selectivity. These ligands can improve the delivery of the PROTAC to the desired tissue, where the recruited E3 ligase will facilitate the degradation process. Additionally, advancements in delivery systems, such as nanoparticles or conjugates, can further improve the tissue-specific delivery of PROTACs.

Furthermore, the identification of novel E3 ligases with restricted tissue distribution is an ongoing area of research. As more ligases are characterized, the repertoire of tissue-specific PROTACs can expand, offering new opportunities for targeted therapy. For instance, the ligases Cereblon (CRBN) and von Hippel-Lindau (VHL) are commonly used in PROTAC design, but exploring other ligases could uncover new targeting mechanisms.

Clinical considerations also play a significant role in the exploitation of tissue-specific ligases. Understanding the dynamics of ligase expression in non-transformed versus diseased tissues can inform the development of PROTACs that are not only selective but also effective in a clinical setting. This requires a careful evaluation of the therapeutic window, dosing strategies, and potential for resistance development.

In summary, the exploitation of tissue-specific ligases for PROTAC delivery is a promising approach that combines molecular biology, biochemistry, and pharmacology. By harnessing the unique expression patterns of E3 ligases, researchers can develop PROTACs that offer targeted degradation of disease-related proteins with high precision. This strategy has the potential to revolutionize the treatment of diseases by providing more effective and safer therapeutic options.

In the realm of PROTAC design, tissue-specific ligases are a critical component for ensuring targeted protein degradation within specific tissues, thereby minimizing systemic toxicity. One prominent example of tissue-specific ligase is MDM2, which is highly expressed in various tumors, including breast, lung, prostate, and gastric cancers. PROTACs that recruit MDM2 have been explored for their potential to selectively degrade oncogenic proteins in these cancer types. Another example is the cereblon (CRBN) ligase, which has been utilized in PROTACs targeting multiple myeloma and other hematologic malignancies due to its expression profile.

The von Hippel-Lindau (VHL) ligase is also frequently employed in PROTAC design, particularly for the degradation of hypoxia-inducible factor (HIF) in renal cell carcinoma, where VHL is often mutated or inactivated. Additionally, the F-box protein β-transducing repeat-containing protein (βTRCP) and the cellular inhibitor of apoptosis (cIAP) have been used in the design of PROTACs for their roles in the ubiquitin-proteasome system and their relevance in certain cancer pathways.

These tissue-specific ligases offer a strategic advantage in PROTAC design by allowing for the selective degradation of disease-causing proteins while sparing healthy tissues. The exploitation of these ligases can lead to more effective and safer therapeutic options for patients. As research progresses, the identification and characterization of additional tissue-specific E3 ligases will likely expand the toolkit available for PROTAC development, potentially leading to breakthroughs in the treatment of a variety of diseases.

PROTACs, or Proteolysis-Targeting Chimeras, are designed to harness the cell's ubiquitin-proteasome system to selectively degrade target proteins. The recruitment of tissue-specific ligases by PROTACs is a critical aspect of their function, allowing for the degradation of proteins within tissues or cells, thereby minimizing systemic side effects. This recruitment is achieved through the careful design of the PROTAC molecule, which consists of two main components: a ligand that binds to the target protein and a ligand that binds to an E3 ubiquitin ligase.

The process begins with the identification of a ligand that has a high affinity for the target protein. This ligand is then linked to another ligand that can bind to an E3 ubiquitin ligase, which is chosen based on its expression in the tissue of interest. The linker between these two ligands is not merely a passive scaffold; its length, composition, and flexibility are meticulously optimized to facilitate the formation of a ternary complex between the PROTAC, the target protein, and the E3 ligase.

Once the ternary complex is formed, the proximity of the E3 ligase to the target protein leads to the transfer of ubiquitin molecules to the target protein, signaling it for degradation by the proteasome. This process effectively removes the target protein from the cell, achieving the therapeutic goal of PROTAC.

The selection of tissue-specific ligases is informed by a detailed understanding of the expression patterns of E3 ligases across different tissues. Some ligases are ubiquitously expressed, while others have more restricted expression profiles, making them ideal for tissue-specific targeting. For example, the von Hippel-Lindau (VHL) ligase is often used in PROTACs targeting renal cell carcinoma, where it is highly relevant due to mutations in the VHL gene.

In addition to the choice of ligase, the design of the PROTAC molecule itself is crucial for ensuring specificity. The ligands must be chosen and positioned in such a way that they do not interfere with the normal function of the E3 ligase but instead redirect its activity towards the target protein. This requires a deep understanding of the structural biology of both the ligase and the target protein.

The development of PROTACs that recruit tissue-specific ligases is a rapidly evolving field, with ongoing research into new ligases and ligands. As our knowledge of the ubiquitin-proteasome system and the role of E3 ligases in various diseases grows, so does the potential for PROTACs to provide targeted treatments for a wide range of conditions.

PROTAC-based therapies, leveraging the mechanism of targeted protein degradation, have shown potential across a broad spectrum of diseases. The versatility of PROTACs lies in their ability to target and degrade proteins that are implicated in disease pathology, making them particularly beneficial for conditions where conventional drugs are ineffective or lack specificity.

Cancer is one of the primary diseases where PROTACs have been extensively studied. They offer a novel approach to targeting and degrading oncoproteins that drive cancer progression, including those previously deemed 'undruggable'. By eliminating these proteins, PROTACs can inhibit tumor growth and proliferation, potentially leading to better clinical outcomes.

Neurodegenerative diseases also stand to benefit from PROTAC technology. Conditions such as Alzheimer's disease, Parkinson's disease, and Huntington's disease are associated with the accumulation of misfolded or aberrant proteins. PROTACs can selectively degrade these pathological proteins, thereby mitigating neurodegeneration and improving neuronal function.

Immune disorders represent another area where PROTACs could have therapeutic applications. By targeting key regulatory proteins within immune signaling pathways, PROTACs can modulate immune responses. This could be particularly useful in autoimmune diseases, where the immune system mistakenly attacks the body's own tissues.

Cardiovascular diseases may also be amenable to PROTAC-based interventions. For instance, PROTACs could target proteins involved in cholesterol metabolism or proteins that contribute to the pathological remodeling of heart tissue following a cardiac event.

Furthermore, PROTACs have been explored for their potential in treating viral infections. By degrading viral proteins or host proteins that viruses hijack for replication, PROTACs could serve as a novel class of antiviral agents. This approach could be especially valuable in the face of emerging viral diseases and drug-resistant strains.

In addition to these diseases, PROTACs have the potential to be applied to a wide range of other conditions. The ongoing discovery and validation of disease-associated proteins as targets for degradation will likely expand the therapeutic scope of PROTACs. As research progresses, PROTACs may become a cornerstone in the treatment of various diseases, offering hope for conditions that have long challenged the medical community.

The development of PROTACs is a dynamic field, with continuous advancements in the design, optimization, and delivery of these molecules. The future of PROTAC-based therapies looks promising, as they hold the potential to transform the landscape of disease treatment by providing highly specific, effective, and potentially safer alternatives to traditional pharmacological interventions.

In the field of cancer treatment, PROTACs (Proteolysis-Targeting Chimeras) have been designed to target a variety of proteins that are critical in the development and progression of cancer. These targeted proteins are often involved in signaling pathways that regulate cell growth, survival, and proliferation, making them key candidates for PROTAC-mediated degradation. For example, ARV-110 is a PROTAC that targets the androgen receptor (AR), which is a significant driver in prostate cancer. By inducing the degradation of AR, ARV-110 aims to inhibit the growth of prostate cancer cells that rely on this receptor for survival.

Another example is ARV-471, which targets the estrogen receptor (ER) in breast cancer. The ER is crucial for the growth of certain types of breast cancer, and its degradation by PROTACs like

ARV-471 can potentially halt the proliferation of these cancer cells. Additionally, FHD-609 is a PROTAC that targets BRD9, a component of the SWI/SNF chromatin remodeling complex implicated in Synovial sarcoma, a rare type of cancer.

Beyond these examples, PROTACs have been developed to target a range of other proteins associated with various cancers. These include BTK (Bruton's tyrosine kinase) in hematologic malignancies, BRD4 (Bromodomain-containing protein 4) in multiple cancer types, CDK-6 (Cyclin-dependent kinase 6) in cell cycle regulation-related cancers, FLT-3 (FMS-like tyrosine kinase-3) in acute myeloid leukemia, HDAC6 (Histone deacetylase 6) in epigenetic regulation of cancer, and STAT3 (Signal transducer and activator of transcription 3) in a variety of cancers including lymphomas and leukemias.

The targeting of these proteins by PROTACs represents a significant advancement in cancer therapy, offering a new strategy to combat the disease by removing key proteins from cancer cells. This approach has the potential to overcome some of the limitations of traditional therapies, such as drug resistance and lack of specificity, by directly targeting the proteins that are essential for cancer cell survival. As research continues, it is likely that more PROTACs targeting a broader range of proteins will be developed, expanding the arsenal of tools available to oncologists for the treatment of cancer. The ongoing clinical trials and studies of PROTACs in cancer treatment are a testament to the potential of this innovative therapeutic strategy to improve outcomes for patients with cancer.

PROTACs (Proteolysis-Targeting Chimeras) represent a novel therapeutic strategy in cancer treatment that differs significantly from traditional small-molecule inhibitors. Traditional small-molecule inhibitors typically function by binding to a protein and inhibiting its activity, which can be effective but often leads to issues such as drug resistance and off-target effects. In contrast, PROTACs are designed to exploit the cell's natural degradation machinery, the ubiquitin-proteasome system, to selectively target and degrade disease-causing proteins.

One of the key advantages of PROTACs over traditional inhibitors is their ability to induce the degradation of target proteins rather than merely inhibiting them. This can lead to a more sustained and complete suppression of the protein's function, potentially resulting in improved therapeutic outcomes. Additionally, because PROTACs act catalytically, a single PROTAC molecule can induce the degradation of multiple target protein molecules, which may allow for lower dosing and reduced side effects.

PROTACs also have the unique ability to target proteins previously considered "undruggable," which are proteins that lack an enzymatic function or a defined active site for a traditional inhibitor to bind. This opens up a vast array of new targets within cancer biology, expanding the potential for treatment options. Moreover, the selectivity of PROTACs can be finely tuned, which helps to minimize the impact on non-target proteins and reduces the likelihood of off-target toxicity.

Another significant benefit of PROTACs is their potential to overcome drug resistance. Cancer cells can develop resistance to traditional inhibitors by mutating the binding site of the drug, rendering the inhibitor ineffective. However, since PROTACs induce protein degradation, they may remain effective even when mutations occur that would typically confer resistance to a traditional inhibitor.

Despite these advantages, PROTACs also face challenges that are being addressed through ongoing research. One of the main challenges is ensuring that PROTACs can effectively penetrate cells and reach their intracellular targets. Additionally, the development of resistance mechanisms to PROTACs themselves, although less common, is a potential concern that requires further investigation.

In summary, PROTACs offer a promising alternative to traditional small-molecule inhibitors in cancer treatment, with the potential for greater efficacy, reduced side effects, and the ability to target a broader range of proteins. As the field of targeted protein degradation continues to evolve, PROTACs may play an increasingly important role in the development of new cancer therapies. The ongoing clinical trials and research into PROTACs will be crucial in determining their place in the future of cancer treatment.

The advancement of PROTACs (Proteolysis-Targeting Chimeras) in clinical settings has been met with several challenges, particularly in achieving tissue-specific delivery. One fundamental issue is ensuring that PROTACs can reach and penetrate the cells of the targeted tissue in sufficient concentrations to exert their therapeutic effects without affecting healthy tissues. This requires a delicate balance of properties such as molecular size, solubility, and stability in the bloodstream. To address these challenges, researchers are exploring various strategies to enhance the tissue-specific delivery of PROTACs.

One approach involves the development of PROTACs that are selective for tissue-specific E3 ligases. By designing PROTACs that recruit these ligases, which are enzymes that catalyze the transfer of ubiquitin to specific substrate proteins, the degradation of proteins can be confined primarily to the target tissue. This strategy leverages the unique expression patterns of E3 ligases across different tissues, allowing for the selective targeting of disease-causing proteins while sparing healthy tissues.

Another strategy is the optimization of the PROTACs' pharmacokinetic (PK) and pharmacodynamic (PD) profiles. These molecules must have a favorable distribution within the body, a suitable half-life to allow for appropriate dosing intervals, and the ability to be metabolized and excreted safely. The inherent physicochemical characteristics of PROTACs, which often include large molecular weights and complex structures due to their bifunctional nature, can impede their ability to diffuse through cell membranes and reach intracellular targets.

Furthermore, the serum stability of PROTACs is crucial for their effectiveness. If a PROTAC is rapidly degraded or inactivated in the bloodstream, it may not reach the target tissue in active form, or it may necessitate higher doses, increasing the risk of side effects. The development of delivery systems that can protect PROTACs from premature degradation while facilitating their release at the target site is an area of ongoing research.

The specificity of E3 ligases, which are integral to the mechanism of action of PROTACs, also poses a challenge. Currently, only a limited number of E3 ligases are utilized in PROTAC design, but the human body has over 600 E3 ligases, some of which are expressed in tissue-specific patterns. Exploiting these tissue-specific ligases could enhance the precision of PROTAC delivery, ensuring that the degradation of target proteins occurs only where needed.

Additionally, the development of resistance to PROTACs is a potential issue. Tumor heterogeneity and the ability of cancer cells to adapt and develop resistance mechanisms could reduce the long-term efficacy of PROTACs. Strategies to overcome resistance may include the design of PROTACs that can target multiple degradation pathways or the combination of PROTACs with other therapeutic agents.

The cellular uptake of PROTACs is another area that requires attention. While some cells may readily internalize these molecules, others may be less permeable, necessitating the development of strategies to enhance cellular uptake, such as the use of cell-penetrating peptides or other delivery vectors.

Lastly, the potential immunogenicity of PROTACs cannot be overlooked. As foreign substances, they may elicit an immune response, which could not only diminish their therapeutic effect but also pose safety concerns. Ensuring that PROTACs are designed to minimize immunogenicity is essential for their successful clinical application.

In conclusion, while PROTACs represent a promising new class of therapeutics with the potential to target previously 'undruggable' proteins, the challenges in their delivery to specific tissues are multifaceted and require innovative solutions. Addressing these challenges is critical for the translation of PROTAC technology from the laboratory to the clinic, where it has the potential to significantly impact the treatment of various diseases.

Enhancing the cellular uptake of PROTACs (Proteolysis-Targeting Chimeras) is a critical step in ensuring their efficacy as therapeutic agents. Several strategies have been developed to improve their delivery into cells. One approach is to modify the physicochemical properties of PROTACs to increase their cell permeability. This can involve altering the molecular weight and polar surface area to facilitate diffusion across the cell membrane. Another strategy is the use of cell-penetrating peptides (CPPs), which are short peptides known to facilitate the transport of cargo molecules into cells. CPPs can be conjugated to PROTACs to improve their intracellular delivery.

Ligand optimization is also a key strategy, where the ligands used for E3 ligase recruitment are modified to enhance their cell permeability. This might include the introduction of hydrophobic groups or the optimization of hydrogen bonding to increase membrane diffusion. Additionally, the linker length and composition between the ligand and the E3 ligase recruiter can be adjusted to improve cellular uptake without compromising the PROTAC's ability to form an effective ternary complex with the target protein and the E3 ligase.

Prodrug strategies are another avenue being explored. In this approach, PROTACs are designed as inactive precursors that can be converted into their active form within the target tissue. This conversion can be triggered by specific enzymes that are present in the target tissue, thereby enhancing the tissue specificity of the PROTAC. Molecular glues, which are small molecules that induce protein-protein interactions, can also be used to improve the cellular uptake of PROTACs. These molecules can enhance the formation of the ternary complex necessary for the ubiquitination and degradation of the target protein.

Nanotechnology-based delivery systems, such as nanoparticles and liposomes, are being investigated to encapsulate PROTACs and protect them from degradation while in circulation. These systems can also be functionalized with targeting ligands to direct the PROTACs to specific tissues or cell types. Furthermore, the use of biomacromolecule-PROTAC conjugates, which combine PROTACs with antibodies, aptamers, or other targeting molecules, can provide a means of enhancing the selectivity and uptake of PROTACs into cells.

Lastly, improving the metabolic stability of PROTACs can also contribute to better cellular uptake. By making PROTACs more resistant to metabolic breakdown, they can remain in circulation longer, increasing the chances of reaching and penetrating target cells. These strategies collectively represent the multifaceted efforts being undertaken to overcome one of the key challenges in the clinical development of PROTACs, ensuring that these promising therapeutic agents can effectively reach and exert their action within diseased cells. As research progresses, it is anticipated that these strategies will continue to evolve and improve, potentially leading to more effective and targeted treatments for a variety of diseases.

PROTACs (Proteolysis-Targeting Chimeras) and other drug delivery systems like nanoparticles and liposomes represent distinct approaches in the delivery of therapeutic agents. PROTACs are bifunctional molecules that induce the degradation of specific target proteins within cells by recruiting the ubiquitin-proteasome system. They are not primarily a delivery system but a therapeutic modality that affects protein levels directly within cells. In contrast, nanoparticles and liposomes are carrier systems designed to improve the delivery and efficacy of drugs, including PROTACs, by enhancing their stability, bioavailability, and targeted delivery to specific tissues or cells.

Nanoparticles, which can be made from a variety of materials including lipids, polymers, and metals, are engineered to carry drugs, including small molecules, proteins, and nucleic acids, to their site of action. They can be designed to release their payload in a controlled manner, potentially reducing the frequency of dosing and side effects. Liposomes, a subset of nanoparticles, are spherical vesicles with a lipid bilayer that can encapsulate drugs, protecting them from degradation in the bloodstream and enhancing their solubility.

The use of nanoparticles and liposomes can address some of the limitations associated with PROTACs, such as poor solubility and stability, potential off-target effects, and the challenge of delivering these larger molecules into cells. By encapsulating PROTACs, these delivery systems can improve their circulation time, reduce immunogenicity, and enhance cellular uptake, which is particularly important given the size and complexity of PROTAC molecules. Moreover, the surface of nanoparticles and liposomes can be modified with targeting ligands, such as antibodies or peptides, to direct the delivery of PROTACs to specific cell types or tissues, thereby increasing their specificity and reducing potential side effects.

However, there are challenges associated with using nanoparticles and liposomes for drug delivery, including the potential for rapid clearance by the immune system, difficulties in manufacturing, and the need to carefully control the release of the drug to avoid toxicity. Additionally, the development of resistance to drug delivery systems, as with any therapeutic approach, is a concern that requires ongoing research.

In summary, while PROTACs offer a novel mechanism of action by targeting the degradation of disease-causing proteins, nanoparticles and liposomes provide a means to enhance the delivery of various therapeutics, including PROTACs. The choice between these approaches depends on the specific therapeutic needs, the nature of the drug being delivered, and the desired outcome. As the field of drug delivery evolves, the integration of PROTACs with advanced delivery systems like nanoparticles and liposomes may lead to more effective and targeted treatments for a range of diseases.

Liposomes, as a drug delivery system, offer a unique set of advantages over other nanoparticle-based systems due to their distinctive composition and characteristics. One of the primary benefits of liposomes is their biocompatibility, as they are composed of phospholipids like those found in cell membranes, which minimizes toxicity and immune responses. This biocompatibility is crucial for reducing adverse effects and ensuring that the drug delivery system is well-tolerated by the body.

Liposomes could encapsulate both hydrophilic and hydrophobic drugs, providing versatility in the types of medications they can deliver. This dual solubility is particularly advantageous for combination therapies, where both types of drugs may be required. Additionally, liposomes can protect the encapsulated drug from degradation in the bloodstream, enhancing the drug's stability and prolonging its half-life. This protection is essential for drugs that are sensitive to enzymatic degradation or have poor stability in biological fluids.

The structure of liposomes allows for controlled release of the drug, which can be tailored to release the drug over a specific period, at a certain rate, or in response to environmental triggers. This controlled release can improve the therapeutic efficacy of the drug and reduce the need for frequent dosing, which enhances patient compliance. Moreover, the size, charge, and surface properties of liposomes can be easily modified, which allows for the optimization of their pharmacokinetic and pharmacodynamic profiles.

Liposomes can also be engineered to target specific tissues or cells by modifying their surface with targeting ligands, such as antibodies or peptides. This targeted delivery can increase the concentration of the drug at the site of action while minimizing exposure to healthy tissues, thereby reducing side effects and improving the therapeutic index. The enhanced permeability and retention (EPR) effect is another advantage of liposomes, where their size allows them to accumulate preferentially in tumor tissues due to the leaky vasculature, further enhancing the targeting of anticancer drugs.

Furthermore, liposomes have been shown to be effective in clinical applications, with several liposomal formulations approved for use in treating diseases such as cancer and fungal infections. Their clinical success underscores their potential and the advantages they offer over other nanoparticle systems. The ability to conjugate various polymers, ligands, and molecules to the liposome structure can improve the effectiveness of anticancer drugs, increasing their sensitivity, specificity, and durability in the body.

In conclusion, liposomes present a multifaceted drug delivery platform with numerous advantages, including biocompatibility, the ability to carry large drug payloads, controlled release mechanisms, and the potential for targeted delivery. These characteristics make liposomes a valuable tool in the field of nanomedicine, particularly for the treatment of complex diseases like cancer, where precision and reduced toxicity are paramount. As research and technology continue to advance, liposomes are likely to play an increasingly significant role in the development of novel therapeutic strategies.

Liposomes and micelles are both lipid-based drug delivery systems that have been extensively used to enhance the therapeutic index of various drugs. Liposomes are vesicular structures composed of phospholipid bilayers that can encapsulate both hydrophilic and hydrophobic drugs within their aqueous core and lipid bilayer, respectively. This dual solubility makes them highly versatile for delivering a range of therapeutic agents. Additionally, liposomes can be engineered to have a prolonged circulation time, which can be beneficial for passive targeting through the enhanced permeability and retention (EPR) effect in tumor tissues.

Micelles, on the other hand, are formed by the self-assembly of amphiphilic molecules in an aqueous solution and typically encapsulate hydrophobic drugs within their core. While micelles are smaller than liposomes, which can be advantageous for certain applications, they generally have a lower drug loading capacity compared to liposomes. However, micelles can be useful for improving the solubility of poorly water-soluble drugs and enhancing their bioavailability.

One of the main differences between liposomes and micelles lies in their structural stability. Liposomes tend to be more stable than micelles, which can disassemble upon dilution in the bloodstream. This stability is crucial for ensuring that the drug remains encapsulated until it reaches the target site. Furthermore, liposomes have been shown to be less prone to clearance by the mononuclear phagocyte system (MPS), which allows for a longer systemic circulation time compared to micelles.

In terms of targeting capabilities, liposomes can be functionalized with ligands such as antibodies or peptides to achieve active targeting to specific cells or tissues. This modification can enhance therapeutic efficacy and reduce side effects by minimizing the impact on non-target tissues. Micelles can also be modified for targeting purposes, but their smaller size and lower stability may limit their effectiveness in some cases.

Both liposomes and micelles have been used in clinically approved formulations, demonstrating their potential as drug delivery systems. However, liposomes have a longer history of clinical use and a broader range of applications, partly due to their higher structural complexity and versatility. The choice between using liposomes or micelles for drug delivery will depend on the specific requirements of the drug, the disease being treated, and the desired pharmacokinetic and pharmacodynamic profiles.

In summary, while both liposomes and micelles offer advantages for drug delivery, liposomes generally provide greater stability, a higher drug loading capacity, and the ability to encapsulate both hydrophilic and hydrophobic drugs. Their ability to be engineered for targeted delivery also makes them a more versatile option for a wide range of therapeutic applications. As research continues, both liposomes and micelles will likely remain important tools in the development of advanced drug delivery systems.

Liposomes and micelles are both lipid-based drug delivery systems that have been extensively used to enhance the therapeutic index of various drugs. Liposomes are vesicular structures composed of phospholipid bilayers that can encapsulate both hydrophilic and hydrophobic drugs within their aqueous core and lipid bilayer, respectively. This dual solubility makes them highly versatile for delivering a range of therapeutic agents. Additionally, liposomes can be engineered to have a prolonged circulation time, which can be beneficial for passive targeting through the enhanced permeability and retention (EPR) effect in tumor tissues.

Micelles, on the other hand, are formed by the self-assembly of amphiphilic molecules in an aqueous solution and typically encapsulate hydrophobic drugs within their core. While micelles are smaller than liposomes, which can be advantageous for certain applications, they generally have a lower drug loading capacity compared to liposomes. However, micelles can be useful for improving the solubility of poorly water-soluble drugs and enhancing their bioavailability.

One of the main differences between liposomes and micelles lies in their structural stability. Liposomes tend to be more stable than micelles, which can disassemble upon dilution in the bloodstream. This stability is crucial for ensuring that the drug remains encapsulated until it reaches the target site. Furthermore, liposomes have been shown to be less prone to clearance by the mononuclear phagocyte system (MPS), which allows for a longer systemic circulation time compared to micelles.

In terms of targeting capabilities, liposomes can be functionalized with ligands such as antibodies or peptides to achieve active targeting to specific cells or tissues. This modification can enhance therapeutic efficacy and reduce side effects by minimizing the impact on non-target tissues. Micelles can also be modified for targeting purposes, but their smaller size and lower stability may limit their effectiveness in some cases.

Both liposomes and micelles have been used in clinically approved formulations, demonstrating their potential as drug delivery systems. However, liposomes have a longer history of clinical use and a broader range of applications, partly due to their higher structural complexity and versatility. The choice between using liposomes or micelles for drug delivery will depend on the specific requirements of the drug, the disease being treated, and the desired pharmacokinetic and pharmacodynamic profiles.

In summary, while both liposomes and micelles offer advantages for drug delivery, liposomes generally provide greater stability, a higher drug loading capacity, and the ability to encapsulate both hydrophilic and hydrophobic drugs. Their ability to be engineered for targeted delivery also makes them a more versatile option for a wide range of therapeutic applications. As research continues, both liposomes and micelles will likely remain important tools in the development of advanced drug delivery systems.

Micelles, as drug delivery systems, are designed to respond to the unique conditions of the tumor microenvironment (TME) to enhance the delivery and efficacy of anticancer drugs. The TME is characterized by a lower pH, higher levels of reactive oxygen species (ROS), and a different redox potential compared to normal physiological conditions. These features are exploited by designing micelles that are sensitive to such stimuli, allowing for a targeted and controlled release of the therapeutic agents they carry.

pH-sensitive micelles are engineered to remain stable in the bloodstream's neutral pH but to disassemble or release their payload in response to the acidic conditions found in tumor tissues. This pH-responsive behavior is typically achieved through the incorporation of acid-labile linkages or groups within the micelle structure that undergo hydrolysis or conformational changes at lower pH levels. As a result, the drug is selectively released in the acidic TME, sparing healthy tissues from exposure and reducing side effects.

Redox-responsive micelles take advantage of the altered redox potential in the TME, where there is an elevated concentration of reducing agents such as glutathione (GSH). These micelles contain disulfide bonds or other redox-sensitive linkages that are stable in the bloodstream but cleave in the presence of high GSH levels, triggering the release of the encapsulated drug. This selective release mechanism ensures that the drug is predominantly released within the tumor, where it can exert its therapeutic action more effectively.

The design of micelles that respond to ROS is another approach to achieve TME-specific drug delivery. In the TME, the concentration of ROS is typically higher than in normal tissues. ROS-responsive micelles are constructed with linkages that are stable under normal conditions but degrade in the presence of ROS, leading to the release of the drug. This strategy not only allows for targeted drug release but also can help to overcome multidrug resistance, a common challenge in cancer treatment.

In addition to these stimuli-responsive designs, micelles can also be engineered to respond to multiple stimuli simultaneously, further refining their specificity and release profiles. For example, dual pH- and redox-responsive micelles can offer a two-step release mechanism, where initial drug release is triggered by the acidic pH of the TME, followed by a secondary release in response to the high redox potential.

Overall, the development of TME-responsive micelles represents a significant advancement in the field of drug delivery. By responding to the specific conditions of the tumor microenvironment, these micelles can improve the precision of drug delivery, enhance the accumulation of drugs at the tumor site, and reduce systemic toxicity. As research in this area continues to progress, it is expected that TME-responsive micelles will play an increasingly important role in the targeted treatment of cancer, offering new hope for patients and contributing to the advancement of precision medicine.

Literatures Cited

Top scientific discoveries and breakthroughs for 2024 | CAS. https://www.cas.org/resources/cas-insights/emerging-science/scientific-breakthroughs-2024-emerging-trends-watch.

Top ten biopharma deals of 2024 - Nature. https://www.nature.com/articles/d43747-024-00027-5.

2024 Predictions: Top Picks | Mass General Brigham. https://www.massgeneralbrigham.org/en/about/newsroom/articles/2024-predictions-top-picks.

Medical breakthroughs and trends you'll hear about in 2024. https://www.scrippsnews.com/science-and-tech/medical-breakthroughs-and-trends-you-ll-hear-about-in-2024.

Microbiology News -- ScienceDaily. https://www.sciencedaily.com/news/plants_animals/microbiology/.

Current Issue: Reviews and Research in Medical Microbiology - LWW. https://journals.lww.com/revmedmicrobiol/Pages/currenttoc.aspx.

Articles | Medical Microbiology and Immunology - Springer. https://link.springer.com/journal/430/articles.

Microbiology News, Research - News-Medical.net. https://www.news-medical.net/?tag=/Microbiology.

Penn uses AI to uncover antibiotics in microbial dark matter. https://www.pennmedicine.org/news/news-releases/2024/june/penn-expert-uses-ai-to-uncover-potential-antibiotics-in-microbial-dark-matter.

Li, M., et al. (2024). Design of a water-soluble transmembrane receptor kinase with intact molecular function by QTY code. Nature Communications. 15, 4293. doi.org/10.1038/s41467-024-48513-9.

About the Author

With a distinguished career as a Medical Microbiologist, having contributed over a hundred research publications to international journals, the impact on the field is substantial. This level of scholarly activity not only advances the understanding of microbial life and its implications for health and disease but also sets a high standard for academic excellence and leadership in the scientific community. The dedication to research and the pursuit of knowledge in this domain are critical in driving innovation and improving clinical outcomes. The insights gained from such extensive research can influence a wide range of areas, from the development of new diagnostic tools and treatments to informing public health policies and strategies. The work of experienced microbiologists is invaluable, particularly in an era where emerging infectious diseases and antibiotic resistance pose significant challenges to global health. The contributions of seasoned researchers help to build a robust body of knowledge that can be leveraged to tackle these issues effectively. Moreover, the mentorship and guidance provided to the next generation of scientists ensure the continued growth and evolution of the field. It's through such prolific research endeavors that medical microbiology continues to evolve, enhancing our ability to respond to the dynamic landscape of infectious diseases and ultimately contributing to the betterment of global health.

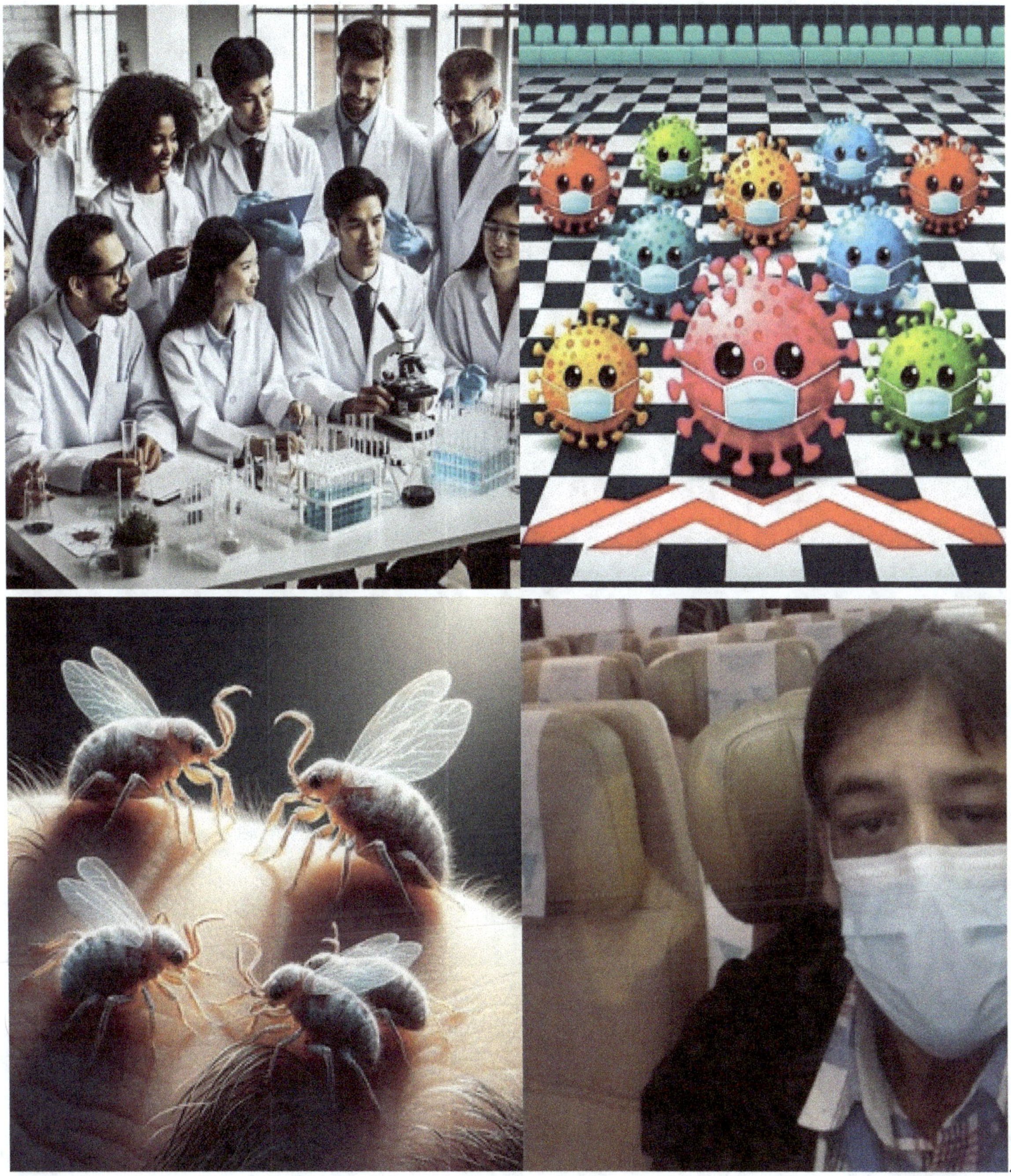

S

arwat Parvez

Maryland, USA